T H E R A

CW00557921

Therapies for diabetes

including oral agents and insulins

Clifford J Bailey
PhD, FRCP(Edin), FRCPath
Head of Diabetes Research
Aston University, Birmingham, UK

Michael D Feher
MB BS, MD, FRCP
Consultant Physician in Diabetes and
Clinical Pharmacology
Chelsea and Westminster Hospital
London, UK

Published by Sherborne Gibbs Limited.
3 Duchess Place, Edgbaston, Birmingham.

© *Sherborne Gibbs Limited 2004*

ISBN: 1-905036-00-0

Printed in the United Kingdom by
Caric Print Limited, Bournemouth, Dorset
in association with Stephens & George Magazines Limited.

PREFACE

This book provides a therapeutic guide for drug treatments used in the management of hyperglycaemia in diabetes mellitus. The topics include the historical background of the drugs and their clinical pharmacology – notably mode of action, indications, efficacy, precautions, interactions, contraindications and adverse effects.

The presentation of concise tables and figures is designed to make therapeutic information readily accessible. It is our hope that this book provides a convenient reference source on current therapies for all members of the multidisciplinary diabetes healthcare team.

Clifford J Bailey
Michael D Feher
2004

CONTENTS

The management of diabetes requires:

- Accurate diagnosis

- Individualised care-plan

- Non-pharmacological life-style measures before and together with drug therapy

Types of diabetes

Diabetes mellitus, characterised by chronic hyperglycaemia, is associated with the risk of developing 'diabetic' microvascular complications (retinopathy, nephropathy and neuropathy) as well as premature macrovascular disease (coronary heart disease, stroke and peripheral vascular disease). These complications are associated with excess morbidity and premature mortality.

Both *impaired fasting glycaemia* and *impaired glucose tolerance* represent a risk of 25 - 50% of developing diabetes over the next 10 years. Impaired glucose tolerance is also associated with premature macrovascular disease (coronary heart disease, stroke and peripheral vascular disease).

Types of diabetes mellitus	
Type 1 diabetes *'insulin-dependent diabetes'* *'ketosis prone diabetes'*	No insulin secretion as a result of the destruction of pancreatic beta-cells (immune-mediated or idiopathic). Insulin is required for survival.
Type 2 diabetes *'non-insulin-dependent diabetes'*	Characterised by disorders of: Insulin secretion and insulin action (either/both features may predominate) Known specific causes of diabetes: Genetic defects of beta-cell function (e.g. MODY syndromes) Genetic defects of insulin action (e.g. leprachaunism) Pancreatic conditions (e.g. pancreatitis) Endocrine conditions (e.g. acromegaly, Cushing's) Drug-induced (steroids, thiazides, beta-blockers)
Gestational diabetes	Diabetes appearing for the first time during pregnancy.

Fig 1.1

Diagnosis of diabetes

Several metabolic conditions characterised by *hyperglycaemia* can be divided into diagnostic categories.

Diagnostic categories		
		Plasma [venous] glucose mmol/L (mg/dL)
Diabetes	Fasting glucose* or	≥7.0 (126)
	Random glucose** or	≥11.1 (200)
	2-hour glucose *during a 75 gm oral glucose tolerance test (OGTT)*	≥11.1 (200)
Impaired Fasting Glycaemia (IFG)	Fasting glucose*	≥6.1 (110), <7.0 (126) *i.e. between 6.1- 6.9*
Impaired Glucose Tolerance (IGT)	2-hour glucose *during a 75 gm oral glucose tolerance test (OGTT)*	≥7.8 (140), <11.1(200)

* *'Fasting': at least 8 hours since last food or energy-containing fluid*
***'Random' is any time of day or night regardless of time of last meal*

Fig 1.2

- Glucose measurement should be repeated in asymptomatic individuals.

- One measurement should be made by a recognised laboratory.

Individualised care-plan and general health education

After comprehensive initial review, which may include referral to several specialties within the multidisciplinary diabetes team, a care-plan should be developed to encompass the general and specific needs of the individual patient.

In addition to initial information about diabetes, advice on diet, exercise and weight control, education on the components of a diabetes care-plan should provide sound practical guidance.

Components of care-plan and practical guidance

Care-plan	Action required to address acute clinical issues identified by initial assessments
	Initial advice on living with diabetes
	Programme of glucose-lowering treatment
	Treatment of associated conditions
	Education programme, including advice on life-style management
	Making contact with other members of care team
	Review schedule and appointments
Practical guidance	Organising a healthy daily routine
	Coping strategies
	Self-monitoring of blood glucose
	Taking medication (including hypoglycaemia)
	Hygiene and avoiding infections
	Recognising and responding to symptoms of common minor intercurrent illness
	Stress reduction measures
	Foot care
	Special occasions (driving, sport, holidays)
	Awareness of complications (including metabolic syndrome)

Fig 1.3

Non-pharmacological life-style management

Advice on life-style management lays the foundation for all programmes of diabetic treatment and includes:

- Diet
- Exercise
- Body weight control
- General health education

Diet

Historical background

Before 1921 (starvation diet)

From 1921 (alterations in diet)

| | | (% Calories) | |
	Carbohydrates	Protein	Fat
1921	20	10	70
1950	40	20	40
1970	45	20	35
1986	up to 60	12 - 20	<30
1994	>55	10 - 15	<30 (Saturated fat <10)

The ideal diet for a person with diabetes is the same as for a normal healthy person. Total amount of energy consumed should be adjusted to achieve and maintain ideal body weight. Frequency and size of meals/snacks will need to be harmonised with daily routine, activity patterns, bouts of exercise, and glucose-lowering drug therapy.

Diet composition: current recommendations

Carbohydrate	>55% of total energy	Added sugar <25 g/day Total sugar <50 g/day
Fat	<30% of total energy	Saturated fat <10% Mono-unsaturated fat 10 - 15% Poly-unsaturated fat <10%
	Fat is 2.25 times more energy dense than carbohydrate or protein, therefore the actual amount of fat consumed should be <15% by weight of the diet	
Cholesterol	<300 mg/day	
Protein	10 - 15% of total energy	
Fibre	>30 g/day	
Salt	<6 g/day	
Alcohol	<30 g/day	

Fig 1.4

- For a total daily energy intake of about 2,000 kcal (8,400 kJ) the amounts of major nutrients should be 280 - 350 g carbohydrate, <70 g fat, and 50 - 70 g protein.

Dietary fibre supplement: guar gum

Guar gum is a soluble fibre supplement which may be used as a dietary adjunct. It is a galactomannan obtained from the Indian cluster bean (*Cyamopsis tetragonoloba*). Although guar gum is used in small amounts as a thickener and stabilising agent in many foods (E412), large amounts are rather unpalatable.

Fig 1.5 Structure of guar gum

Guar gum at a glance

Action	Soluble dietary fibre supplement
Clinical effects	1. Reduction of hyperglycaemia 2. Lowering of postprandial insulin concentrations in type 2 diabetes 3. Reduction in LDL-cholesterol (small effect)
Indication	• *Type 2 diabetes*
Usage	Guar gum with main meals can reduce postprandial hyperglycaemia by delaying digestion/absorption of dietary carbohydrate
Treatment	Guar gum is available in 5 g sachets – normally added to ~200 ml of fluid taken with meal: alternatively, contents of sachet can be sprinkled on food, provided there is plenty of fluid to accompany meal Since guar swells on contact with liquid, it is better to consume with fluid
Contraindications	History of gastrointestinal obstruction, oesophageal disease or dysphagia
Adverse effects	Abdominal distention and flatulence
Precautions	Taken without adequate fluid, the swelling of guar gum in the gut may cause obstruction Large amounts are rather unpalatable Guar gum should not be considered as an alternative to a healthy diet already rich in fibre

Exercise

Aerobic physical activity should be encouraged with appropriate regard to contraindications, capabilities and inclination of the patient.

Realistic aerobic exercises for a previously sedentary adult – aim to build up to:

- Brisk walking >15 min
- Jogging >10 min
- Cycling >15 min
- Swimming >10 min (especially if unsuited to other exercises)
- Gardening or housework

Principles and effects of exercise	
Principles of exercise	Building up gradually
	Set realistic targets
	Harmonisation with diet and drug therapy
	Awareness of hypoglycaemia
	Awareness of foot care
Physiological effects	Glucose utilisation due to increased insulin sensitivity
	Insulin-independent effects of muscle contraction

Fig 1.6

Body weight control

An important part of therapy is to achieve and maintain ideal body weight.

Clinical assessments of weight		
Body Mass Index (BMI)		
$BMI = weight (kg)/height (metres)^2$ (kg/m^2)	*World Health Organisation (WHO) classification of overweight and obesity*	
		BMI
	Underweight	<18.5
	Normal	18.5 - 24.9
	Overweight	25 - 29.9
	Obese	≥30
	Extreme obesity	≥40
Waist circumference (Waist)	*Men*	94 cm (37 in)
For Europids	*Women*	88 cm (34.5 in)
Waist-to-hip ratio (WHR)	*Men*	>0.95
For Europids	*Women*	>0.80

Fig 1.7

Categories of Body Mass Index (BMI), kg/m^2

Weight (lbs)

Height (feet and inches)	110	120	130	140	150	160	170	180	190	200	210	220	230	240	250	Height (metres)
4'10"	23	25	27	29	31	33	36	38	40	42	44	46	48	50	52	1.47
4'11"	22	24	26	28	30	32	34	36	38	40	42	44	47	49	51	1.50
5'0"	21	23	25	27	29	31	33	35	37	39	41	43	45	47	49	1.52
5'1"	20	23	25	26	28	30	32	34	36	38	40	42	43	46	47	1.55
5'2"	20	22	24	26	27	29	31	33	35	37	39	40	42	44	46	1.57
5'3"	19	21	23	25	27	28	30	32	34	36	38	39	41	43	44	1.60
5'4"	19	21	22	24	26	27	29	31	33	35	37	38	39	41	43	1.63
5'5"	18	20	22	23	25	27	28	30	32	34	36	37	38	40	42	1.65
5'6"	18	19	21	23	24	26	27	29	31	33	35	36	37	39	40	1.68
5'7"	17	19	20	22	23	25	27	28	30	32	34	35	36	38	39	1.70
5'8"	17	18	20	21	23	24	26	27	29	31	33	34	35	36	38	1.73
5'9"	16	18	19	21	22	24	25	27	28	30	32	33	34	35	37	1.75
5'10"	16	17	19	20	22	23	24	26	27	29	31	32	33	34	36	1.78
5'11"	15	17	18	20	21	22	24	25	26	28	30	31	32	33	35	1.80
6'0"	15	16	18	19	20	22	23	24	26	27	29	30	31	33	34	1.83
6'1"	15	16	17	18	20	21	22	24	25	26	28	29	30	32	33	1.85
6'2"	14	16	17	18	19	21	22	23	24	26	27	28	30	31	32	1.87
	50	55	59	64	68	73	77	82	86	91	95	100	105	109	114	

Weight (kg)

Underweight　Normal　Overweight　Obese

Fig 1.8

Weight management: underweight

In underweight diabetic patients, especially children, high protein low fat enteral food supplements can be helpful during:

- Intercurrent illness, or
- In individuals who cannot or will not take normal meals, or
- In individuals who persistently fail to thrive

Weight management: overweight and obese

Reducing adiposity improves glycaemic control through increased insulin sensitivity. The reductions in weight are associated with improvements in both the dyslipidaemia and hypertension that often accompany obesity.

Management of overweight and obese individuals

Diet modification

Clinical aspects	Reducing total daily energy intake is usually the most effective means of weight loss. *Care must be taken to avoid loss of lean body mass.*
	Supervised use of energy-restricted diets should focus on a reduction of saturated fat content of diet while ensuring adequate consumption of vitamins, minerals, fibre and protein.
	Non-nutritive sweeteners and dietary 'bulking' agents can be useful.
Compliance	Notoriously poor.

Anti-obesity drugs

Use	Adjunct to diet, exercise and health education to assist loss of excess adipose tissue.
Mode of action	*Orlistat* – inhibits fat digestion *Sibutramine* – acts mainly by inducing satiety
Effects	Weight loss of 2 - 3 kg, occasionally >5 kg, greater than by non-pharmacological measures. *This is less weight loss than usually seen in non-diabetic individuals.*
	About twice as many diabetic individuals achieve significant weight loss with these drugs: *Approximately 50% achieve >5% weight loss, compared with about 25% of patients on non-pharmacological treatment alone.*
	Weight loss of 5 - 10% may be accompanied by reduction of up to 1% in HbA1c.
Compliance	Notoriously poor.

Fig 1.9

Orlistat at a glance

Action	Pancreatic lipase inhibitor acting in the intestinal lumen to reduce fat digestion which in turn reduces fat absorption
Indications	• Obese (BMI $\geq$30 kg/m^2) • Overweight (BMI $\geq$28 kg/m^2) +co-morbidity *e.g. type 2 diabetes, hypertension, dyslipidaemia*
Pre-treatment	Weight loss $\geq$2.5 kg achieved in 4 weeks by non-pharmacological measures (diet and exercise)
Usage	Adjunct to non-pharmacological measures
Treatment	Start 120 mg immediately before, with or up to 1 hour after the main meal(s), titrate up to maximum 360 mg daily Maximum treatment period 2 years *Discontinue if weight loss <5% initial body weight at 3 months or <10% initial body weight at 6 months*
Contraindications	Chronic malabsorption syndrome Cholestasis Pregnancy, breast-feeding
Adverse effects	Loose fatty stools, oily evacuation Abdominal discomfort Flatulence Increased defecation, occasionally faecal incontinence
Precautions	Side-effects minimised by reducing fat content of meals Possible reduced absorption of fat-soluble vitamins, therefore advise taking a once-daily multivitamin supplement Not recommended in children (<18 years) and elderly (>75 years) Avoid concomitant use with acarbose

Sibutramine at a glance

Action	Centrally acting satiety inducer: also maintains thermogenic energy expenditure Inhibits reuptake of serotonin and noradrenaline

Indications	• Obese (BMI $\geq$30 kg/m²)
	• Overweight (BMI $\geq$27 kg/m²)
	   + co-morbidity *e.g. type 2 diabetes,*
	               dyslipidaemia

Pre-treatment	Failure to achieve weight loss of 5% of initial weight after serious attempt by non-pharmacological measures (diet, exercise and health education) for $\geq$3 months
Usage	Adjunct to non-pharmacological measures
Treatment	Start 10 mg o.d. in the morning, increase to 15 mg o.d. if weight loss <2 kg at 4 weeks Maximum treatment period 1 year *Discontinue if 15 mg o.d. does not produce weight loss $\geq$2 kg at 4 weeks or $\geq$5% initial body weight at 3 months or there is weight regain $\geq$3 kg of previous weight loss*
Contraindications	Inadequately controlled hypertension Severe hepatic or renal disease Serious eating disorders or psychiatric illness Existing or previous cardiovascular disease Monoamine oxidase inhibitor, alcohol abuse Narrow angle glaucoma, hyperthyroidism Pregnancy, breast-feeding Previous hypersensitivity to sibutramine
Adverse effects	Increased blood pressure (BP) and heart rate (HR), dry mouth, anorexia, constipation, insomnia, asthenia
Precautions	Monitor BP and HR frequently *e.g. measure BP every 2 weeks for first 3 months* Not recommended in children and elderly Possible interactions with other centrally acting drugs, erythromycin and ketoconozole, and drugs that are highly protein-bound Likely to enhance blood glucose-lowering effect of glucose-lowering drugs

2 PRINCIPLES OF GLUCOSE-LOWERING DRUG THERAPY

The main aims of treatment of diabetes include:

- Save life

- Optimise glycaemic control

  The primary aim of therapy is to improve glycaemic control to as near normal (normoglycaemia) as possible.

- Alleviate symptoms

- Prevent microvascular and macrovascular complications

  Improved glycaemic control can delay or prevent the onset and reduce the severity of microvascular complications, with benefits continuing to accrue until normoglycaemia is reinstated.

  Improved glycaemic control reduces the risk of macrovascular complications which are often associated with the metabolic syndrome (insulin resistance syndrome), of which hyperglycaemia is a component.*

Glucose-lowering drug therapy

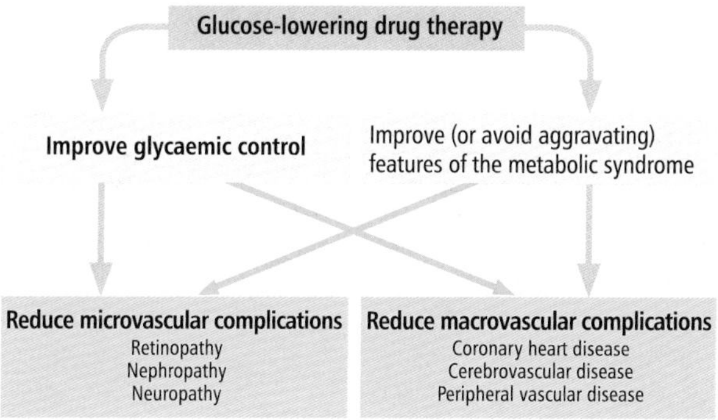

Fig 2.1

---

* metabolic syndrome *comprises:*
insulin resistance, hyperinsulinaemia, abdominal obesity, dyslipidaemia (raised serum triglyceride, increased proportion of small dense LDL, low HDL-cholesterol), raised blood pressure, hyperglycaemia, pro-coagulant state, and is associated with atherosclerosis.

Treatment algorithms

All drug therapies for diabetes should be regarded as adjuncts to non-pharmacological measures which should be reviewed and reinforced as part of ongoing management.

Type 1 diabetes

● Initiate insulin therapy immediately *(see Chapter 8), selecting and intensifying the regimen tailored to the individual patient.*

Type 2 diabetes

● Treatment of type 2 diabetes is complex and requires an individualised, flexible and adaptable approach.

Treatment algorithm: type 2 diabetes

Diagnosis

Non-pharmacological measures
Diet, exercise, weight control, health education

Move to next stage if desired glycaemic control not achieved

Oral monotherapy
Metformin, thiazolidinedione*,
sulphonylurea, meglitinide, acarbose

Oral combination therapy
Two differently acting agents from monotherapy
list, or add thiazolidinedione**

Insulin
With/without an oral agent†

* Thiazolidinedione monotherapy if metformin inappropriate (Europe)

** Triple oral therapy using 3 differently acting oral agents is not recommended in the UK, but may be appropriate to achieve desired glycaemic control, or to maintain glycaemic control while changing the combination of oral agents

† Introduction of insulin may involve continuing one or more oral agents

Fig 2.2

Individualised tailored therapy in type 2 diabetes is required:

- Presentation is highly variable
- Treatment must be harmonised with life-style
- Natural history of the disease is progressive (rate and nature of progression are highly variable)
- Various concurrent medical conditions usually exist (often requiring multiple medications)

The treatment process begins with non-pharmacological measures which should be reinforced in conjunction with pharmacological therapies.

Monotherapy with one oral agent is tried first. If this does not achieve or maintain adequate glycaemic control then a *combination* of two (and occasionally three) differently acting oral agents is used.

If these do not achieve or maintain adequate glycaemic control, then *insulin therapy* is commenced, with or without continuation of one or two oral agents.

Additional point

1. Patients with severe beta-cell failure, which is typically indicated by marked and escalating hyperglycaemia with unintentional weight loss, are unlikely to respond adequately to any oral agents. These patients should be treated with insulin.

Summary of glucose-lowering drugs	
Class	**Main action**
Biguanide *(Metformin)*	Counter insulin resistance *(multiple actions)*
Sulphonylurea	Increase insulin secretion *(slower and longer acting than meglitinide)*
Meglitinide	Increase insulin secretion *(faster and shorter acting than sulphonylurea)*
Thiazolidinedione	Increase insulin sensitivity *(PPARγ agonists)*
α-Glucosidase inhibitor *(Acarbose)*	Decrease intestinal carbohydrate digestion
Insulin	Physiological effects of insulin *(decrease hepatic glucose output, increase peripheral glucose uptake)*

Fig 2.3

Targets for glycaemic control

Glycaemic control is the principal gauge for diabetes therapies.
It is also the main metabolic parameter to monitor and is determined by:

● Fasting plasma glucose
● HbA1c
● Self-monitoring (by patient) of capillary blood glucose

Management of diabetes also requires management of other factors relevant to the metabolic syndrome (especially blood pressure and lipids), potential contraindications for drug therapy and drug interactions, and any other aspects of treatment that could influence microvascular, neuropathic and macrovascular complications.

Treatment targets for diabetes		
	'Optimum'	**'Audit standard'**
Glycaemia		
HbA1c	<6.5%	<7.5% (NICE guidelines)
Fasting glucose	*mmol/L (mg/dL)*	*mmol/L (mg/dL)*
venous	≤6.0 (110)	≤6.5 (118)
capillary†	≤5.5 (100)	≤6.0 (110)
Lipids*	*mmol/L (mg/dL)*	*mmol/L (mg/dL)*
Total-cholesterol	<4.0 (155)	<5.0 (193)
LDL-cholesterol	<2.0 (77)	<3.0 (115)
HDL-cholesterol	>1.2 (46)	>1.0 (39)
Serum triglycerides	<1.7 (150)	<2.2 (195)
Blood pressure		
BP (SBP/DBP) *seated*	130/80 mmHg	140/80 mmHg
Body weight		
BMI (kg/m²)	19 - 25	
Waist-to-hip ratio	<0.95 *Men*	
	<0.80 *Women*	
	† *Fasting capillary blood glucose is about 1 mmol/L (18 mg/dL) lower than fasting venous plasma glucose*	
	* *Fasting*	

Fig 2.4

Additional points

1. These targets are not always attainable, or indeed desirable, in all patients or all circumstances e.g. elderly, infirm, drivers.
2. 'Moderate control' has been defined by European Diabetes Policy Group (*Diabetic Medicine* 1999, **16:** 716-730), however these less rigid targets may leave patients at higher risk of complications.

Methods of glucose monitoring

Details of method	Use in clinical practice

HbA1c

Measures the non-enzymatic attachment of glucose to haemoglobin A1c which is an indicator of overall glycaemia during the previous 6 - 8 weeks.

Long-term glycaemic control is most usefully assessed by the percentage of glycated haemoglobin A1c (HbA1c).

Check HbA1c every 2 - 6 months.

Reference standard range for non-diabetic individuals: HbA1c 4 - 6%

Target for optimal glycaemic control in diabetes: HbA1c <6.5% (European Policy Group)

Fructosamine

Assay of glycated plasma proteins, mainly non-enzymatic attachment of glucose to albumin. Indicates overall glycaemia during the previous 2 - 3 weeks.

As there is no recognised inter-laboratory standardisation of the assay it is not widely used.

Plasma glucose (venous)

Most assays are based on glucose oxidase or hexokinase method.

Most widely used measure of short-term glycaemic control for titrating the dosage of drugs.

Fasting glucose should be ≤6 mmol/L (110 mg/dL) to retain the safety margin against hypoglycaemia *(preferably not below 5 mmol/L [90 mg/dL])*.

Self-monitoring of (capillary) blood glucose

Solid phase glucose oxidase or hexokinase with colorimetric or amperometric measurement.

Most finger-stick blood glucose meters are calibrated to give a venous plasma equivalent value. These are accurate for use by healthcare professionals and patients.

Self-monitoring of blood glucose should be encouraged for all patients where practicable. *Frequency will be greater during drug dose adjustment, unstable control or irregular life-styles.* Under stable conditions, self-monitoring is recommended on at least one day per week.

Capillary glucose control (mmol/L)

	Desirable	Moderate
Before breakfast	4 - 6	<7
1 - 2 h after main meal	<8	<10

Patients taking insulin or oral insulin-releasing agents are advised to measure blood glucose whenever they experience symptoms of hypoglycaemia that are more than very mild and are not relieved by a small amount of oral glucose or other snack.

Fig 2.5

Starting oral glucose-lowering drug therapy

Whether starting monotherapy or adding another drug for combination therapy, a key treatment principle is to achieve optimal glycaemic control using the lowest effective amount of drug administered in the most convenient manner.

Starting oral drug therapy	
Factors for drug selection	Pathophysiological status Life-style Co-existent conditions and medications Desired level of control Contraindications and precautions
1. Start with a low dose	*Once-daily* (usually with breakfast) for an intermediate or long-acting agent or *Twice-daily* (usually with breakfast and with mid-day or early evening meal) for a short-acting agent *Patient should self-monitor blood glucose before breakfast and 1 - 2 h after a main meal on at least two days per week during initial 1 - 2 weeks.*
2. Increase dosage	If desired control or substantial reduction in blood glucose is not observed by 2 - 4 weeks. *For most drugs, titration steps are at about 2 week intervals.* *Some agents (e.g. thiazolidinediones) have a slow onset of efficacy, and titration steps may be at 4 - 8 week intervals.*
3. Continue to monitor glycaemic control	As dosage increases, it may be appropriate to use intermediate or long-acting drugs in divided doses. *Increase vigilance for interprandial and nocturnal hypoglycaemia and drug interactions.*
• If dosage is increased without improvement in glycaemic control over 4 weeks of treatment	Return to the previous dosage level.
• If glycaemic control is not satisfactory with maximum effective dosage	With monotherapy – add a second oral agent or if already taking two oral agents, commence insulin or *if already taking two oral agents add a third oral agent** *(* only in selected clinical circumstances)*

Fig 2.6

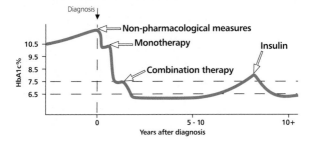

Typical changes of HbA1c during treatment: type 2 diabetes

Fig 2.7

Additional points

1. In newly diagnosed type 2 diabetes, when non-pharmacological measures and one oral agent do not achieve adequate glycaemic control, it is appropriate to consider combination therapy without delay.

2. If an adult patient presents with severe hyperglycaemia (e.g. fasting plasma glucose >12 mmol/L or HbA1c >10%) it is likely that combination therapy will be required.

3. Some adults who present with very severe hyperglycaemia may already have a sufficiently marked loss of beta-cell function that insulin should be initiated.

4. In type 2 patients who have previously achieved satisfactory control with two oral agents but whose control is deteriorating (often with unintentional weight loss), insulin therapy is indicated.

Treatment changes with severe illness and surgery in type 2 diabetes	
Condition	**Management**

Severe intercurrent illness
Myocardial infarction
Severe infection and shock
Hospital admission for:
  – Major/elective surgery
  – Highly debilitating illness
  – Malnutrition
  – Pregnancy
	Temporarily stop oral therapy and institute insulin therapy

Fig 2.8

3 ALPHA-GLUCOSIDASE INHIBITORS

Historical background

1991   Acarbose, first alpha-glucosidase inhibitor used in clinical practice.

    – Acarbose is the only member of this class used in the UK.

    – Miglitol and voglibose are used in some countries.

Fig 3.1 Structure of acarbose

Alpha-glucosidase inhibitors act mainly to lower postprandial hyperglycaemia by slowing the rate of carbohydrate digestion.

The lower postprandial glycaemic peak during use in type 2 diabetes is generally associated with lower postprandial insulin concentrations.

Overall, the modest efficacy and gastrointestinal side-effects have limited use of acarbose in the UK.

Acarbose: pharmacokinetics

Acarbose: pharmacokinetics	
Bioavailability	Site of action – intestine (~100% bioavailable)
Absorption	<2% of an oral dose is absorbed as intact drug
	~30% absorbed as intestinal metabolites
Metabolism	~50% metabolised (degraded) by intestinal amylases and bacteria
Elimination	Unabsorbed drug and metabolites eliminated in faeces
	Absorbed drug and metabolites eliminated in urine within 24 hours without any systemic effects

Fig 3.2

Acarbose: mode of action

- Slows the digestion of complex carbohydrates and sucrose in the small intestine

- Competitively inhibits the activity of alpha-glucosidase enzymes

  The enzymes (glucoamylase, maltase, dextrinase and sucrase) are localised in the brush border membranes of enterocytes lining the intestinal villi (Fig 3.3). Acarbose binds to these enzymes with much greater affinity than their natural disaccharide and oligosaccharide substrates. Thus acarbose prevents these alpha-glucosidase enzymes from cleaving off the absorbable monosaccharides.

- Acarbose also causes a modest inhibition of alpha-amylase activity

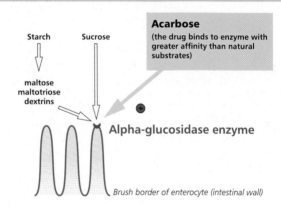

Mechanism of alpha-glucosidase inhibition

Starch Sucrose

Acarbose
(the drug binds to enzyme with greater affinity than natural substrates)

maltose
maltotriose
dextrins

Alpha-glucosidase enzyme

Brush border of enterocyte (intestinal wall)

Fig 3.3

The effectiveness of acarbose is dependent, therefore, on administration of the drug together with a meal rich in complex carbohydrate. Acarbose prolongs the period of carbohydrate digestion and defers the process further along the intestinal tract. This in turn delays and extends the period of glucose absorption, which lowers the height of the postprandial glucose excursion, and prolongs its duration.

Acarbose: indications		
Type 2 diabetes *obese and non-obese*	First-line monotherapy *when there is inadequate glycaemic control by non-pharmacological measures.*	Most suited to monotherapy are those with minimal basal hyperglycaemia but more pronounced postprandial hyperglycaemia.
	Second-line drug therapy *when monotherapy with these agents plus non-pharmacological measures do not achieve adequate glycaemic control.*	In combination with: – Metformin – Meglitinide – Sulphonylurea – Insulin Useful with persistent postprandial hyperglycaemia despite control of basal glycaemia.
Type 1 diabetes	Combination with insulin *when an optimal insulin regimen together with non-pharmacological measures do not achieve adequate glycaemic control.*	Useful with persistent postprandial hyperglycaemia despite control of basal glycaemia.

Fig 3.4

Acarbose: starting therapy

- Acarbose should always be **taken with meals** that are rich in complex carbohydrate: patient education and compliance are essential.

- The tablets can either be chewed or swallowed whole at the start of the meal.

- Start with a low dose (e.g. 50 mg with one main meal), then increase over 1 - 4 weeks to 50 mg with each of two or three main meals daily. Monitor postprandial glycaemic control by patient self-monitoring at 1 hour or 2 hours after beginning the meal. Also check fasting glucose values.

- Continue to increase the dosage slowly over 4 - 8 weeks up to 100 mg with each of three main meals. This is the maximum recommended dose, but a higher dosage of 200 mg with each main meal can be used if the extra dosage continues to benefit glycaemic control and is tolerated.

Acarbose: efficacy

- Since acarbose delays carbohydrate digestion, the predominant effect on glycaemic control is to reduce the height of postprandial hyperglycaemia. The period of glucose absorption is also extended (Fig 3.5). This tends to create a smoother day-profile of blood glucose, and can reduce interprandial troughs of hypoglycaemia.

- Given as monotherapy to patients who comply adequately with dietary advice, acarbose can reduce peak postprandial glucose by 1 to 4 mmol/L. The 0 - 2 hour postprandial increment in blood glucose can be halved by acarbose, although the effect is generally smaller as glycaemic control approaches the normal range.

- There is a small carry-over from the postprandial effect of acarbose to reduce basal glycaemia. During chronic therapy fasting plasma glucose may decrease by up to 1 mmol/L.

- The decrease in HbA1c is usually about 0.5%, but can be >1% in patients with substantial postprandial hyperglycaemia who receive high dose acarbose monotherapy and show dietary compliance. Similar efficacy can be achieved when acarbose is added to another antidiabetic agent.

Additional points

1. Acarbose can have a trivial effect on the absorption of other oral hypoglycaemic agents without any clinical effect.

2. Acarbose does not cause weight gain and may produce a small lowering of postprandial insulin and triglyceride concentrations.

3. The safety record of acarbose is good provided contraindications are respected.

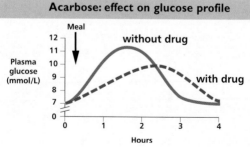

Fig 3.5

Acarbose: adverse effects

Gastrointestinal side-effects

Generalised abdominal discomfort and sometimes diarrhoea.

Initially this is due to the dosage being increased too rapidly. If symptoms persist the dosage may be too great relative to the amount of complex carbohydrate in the diet, such that undigested oligosaccharides pass into the large bowel. Here they are fermented by bacteria, causing flatulence, soft stools, meteorism, borborygmi.

Since these events are most common during initiation of the treatment, dosage should be titrated slowly.

Most of these events resolve with a reduction in dosage and slower titration, and usually subside with time.

Hypoglycaemia

Not a problem with acarbose monotherapy.

Acarbose in combination with insulin or an insulin-releasing agent (sulphonylurea or meglitinide) can sometimes *precipitate or aggravate hypoglycaemic episodes.* However, by extending the period of carbohydrate digestion acarbose is more likely to reduce interprandial hypoglycaemia.

Because acarbose delays digestion of sucrose, it is important to take glucose (not sucrose) to combat any hypoglycaemic symptoms.

Liver damage

Highest doses have been associated in isolated cases.

Fig 3.6

Acarbose: precautions, interactions, contraindications

Precautions

Periodic checks – renal function (e.g. serum creatinine).
      – liver function (e.g. serum alanine transaminase), especially if the dosage of acarbose is high.

Drug interactions

None significant.

Cholestyramine slightly enhances the glucose-lowering effect of acarbose.

Agents affecting gut motility could potentially alter the effectiveness and GI side-effects of acarbose.

Contraindications

Severe renal and liver disease.

History of chronic intestinal disorders.

Pregnancy, breast-feeding and children under 12 years old (although no special problems are known).

Fig 3.7

Acarbose at a glance

Class	Alpha-glucosidase inhibitor
Action	Slows carbohydrate digestion which reduces the rise in postprandial hyperglycaemia

Indications[*]	• *Type 2 diabetes*
	  – Monotherapy
	  – Combination with other oral glucose-lowering drugs or insulin
	• *Type 1 diabetes*
	  – Combination with insulin

Dosage form	Tablets 50 mg, 100 mg (scored)
Treatment	Patient education to take with meals rich in complex carbohydrate Start 50 mg with one main meal – Titrate slowly to 50 mg each main meal – Titrate slowly to 100 mg each main meal Maximum recommended dose 3 x 100 mg daily
Contraindications	Severe renal and liver disease History of chronic intestinal disease
Efficacy	HbA1c ↓0.5 - 1.0% Postprandial glycaemia ↓1 - 4 mmol/L
Adverse effects	Gastrointestinal disturbances, especially flatulence Very rarely abnormal liver function
Precautions	Periodic check of serum creatinine and liver enzymes if using high doses Possible hypoglycaemia when used with other glucose-lowering drugs

[*] Indication assumes inadequate glycaemic control with non-pharmacological measures (and existing pharmacological therapy for combination use)

Historical background

1942	Loubatieres observed/sulphonamide-induced hypoglycaemia.
1946	Janbon reported sulphonamide group essential for glucose-lowering.
1955	Carbutamide – a sulphonylurea – assessed clinically.
1950s-60s	1st generation sulphonylureas (*tolbutamide* and *chlorpropamide*) introduced into clinical practice.
Late 1960s-90s	2nd generation sulphonylureas (*glibenclamide, glipizide, gliclazide* and *glimepiride*) introduced.
1970	Universities Group Diabetes Program (UGDP) – first major outcome trial of sulphonylurea treatment.
1998	United Kingdom Prospective Diabetes Study (UKPDS) – second major outcome trial of sulphonylurea treatment.

Sulphonylureas act on the pancreatic beta-cells to stimulate insulin secretion, provided there is adequate beta-cell function. The extra insulin secretion reduces basal and postprandial hyperglycaemia.

The main side-effect is hypoglycaemia.

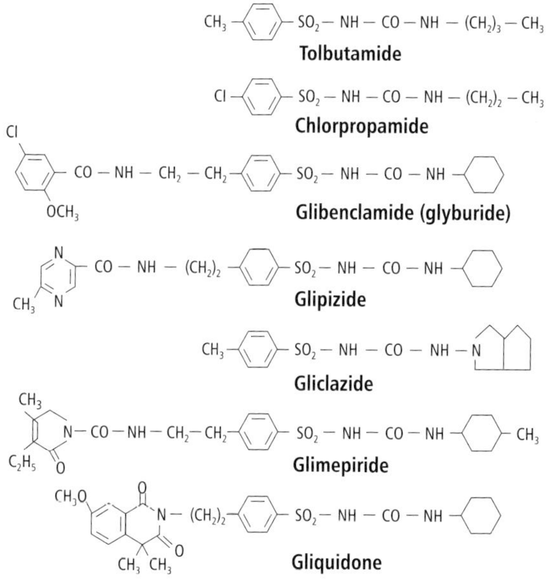

Fig 4.1 Structure of sulphonylureas

Sulphonylureas: pharmacokinetics

The different structures of sulphonylureas provide a range of pharmacokinetic properties which include wide variations in hepatic metabolism, activity of metabolites, and route and time of elimination. These features affect the duration of action from *short* (<12 h) to *long* (>24 h).

- *Low binding affinity* is a feature of **1st generation sulphonylureas** – therefore given in large milligram doses. *Greater binding properties* from additional chemical moieties of the **2nd generation sulphonylureas** allow usage in lower doses.
- Almost all of an oral dose of all sulphonylureas is absorbed.
- Peak plasma concentration in 2 - 4 hours.
- All highly protein-bound – potential for interaction with other highly protein-bound drugs.

	Duration of action (hours)	Time to peak plasma concentration (hours)	Protein-bound
Tolbutamide	6 - 10	3 - 4	>95%
Glipizide	6 - 16	1 - 3	~98%
Gliquidone	6 - 18	2 - 3	~99%
Gliclazide	12 - 20	2 - 4	>85%
Gliclazide MR	~24	4 - 12	>87%
Glimepiride	12 - >24	2 - 3	>99%
Glibenclamide	12 - >24	2 - 4	>98%
Chlorpropamide	24 - 50	2 - 4	~95%

Sulphonylureas

Fig 4.2A

Sulphonylureas: pharmacokinetics

		Daily dosage (mg)	Duration of action[a]	Activity of metabolites	Metabolites	Elimination t½ (hours)	Elimination
Tolbutamide	1st generation	500 - 2,000	Short	Inactive	Hydroxy- Carboxy-	4 - 7 [28][a]	Urine 100%
Glipizide	2nd generation	2.5 - 20	Short-intermediate	Inactive	Hydroxy- Others	2 - 7	Urine ~70%
Gliquidone	2nd generation	15 - 180	Short-intermediate	Inactive	Hydroxy-	2 - 8 [24][a]	Bile ~65%
Gliclazide	2nd generation	40 - 320	Intermediate	Inactive	Demethy-	6 - 14 [20][a]	Urine ~65%
Gliclazide MR	2nd generation	30 - 120	Intermediate-long	Inactive	Hydroxy- Carboxy- ~6 others	~17	Urine ~65%
Glimepiride	2nd generation	1 - 6	Intermediate-long	Active	Hydroxy- Carboxy-	5 - 9 [~24][a]	Urine ~60%
Glibenclamide	2nd generation	2.5 - 15	Intermediate-long	Active	Hydroxy- Others	10 - 20 [>24][a]	Bile >50%
Chlorpropamide	1st generation	100 - 500	Long	Active	Hydroxy- Chlorobenzyl	24 - 50	Urine >90%

[a]Short <12 h; Intermediate 12 - 24 h; Long 18 - >24 h.

Gliclazide MR (Diamicron MR) is a modified release formulation: 30 mg of the MR formulation is approximately therapeutically equivalent to 80 mg of standard gliclazide

Fig 4.2B

[Metabolites][a]

Sulphonylureas: mode of action

Pancreatic
(main effect)

1. Stimulate insulin secretion.

2. Initiate insulin secretion at low glucose concentrations (hence risk of hypoglycaemia).

3. Enhance glucose-stimulated insulin release.

Dependent on functional pancreatic beta-cells in the islets of Langerhans.
Drug binds to sulphonylurea (SUR-1) receptors in plasma membrane of beta-cells.
[SUR-1 is part of the ATP-sensitive potassium channels (K^+-ATP channels)](Fig 4.4).

Mechanism

→ *Closure of K^+-ATP channels reduces potassium efflux.*
→ *Local intracellular retention of potassium causes membrane depolarisation which opens voltage-dependent calcium influx channels.*
→ *Rise in intracellular free calcium concentration activates calcium-dependent proteins with release (exocytosis) of insulin granules.*

Extra-pancreatic
(weak effect)

1. Reduce hepatic glucose output.
2. Potentiate peripheral insulin-mediated glucose uptake.

It is uncertain whether these extra-pancreatic effects are clinically significant at therapeutic concentrations.

Fig 4.3

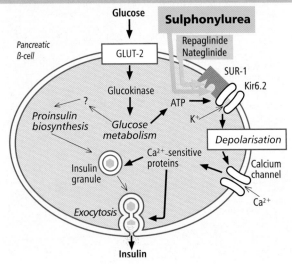

Mechanism of insulin release by sulphonylureas

Fig 4.4

Sulphonylureas: indications

Since sulphonylureas may cause weight gain, they are generally used in non-obese/overweight individuals.

Sulphonylureas: indications		
Type 2 diabetes non-obese or obese	First-line monotherapy *when there is inadequate glycaemic control by non-pharmacological measures.*	
	Second-line drug therapy *when monotherapy with other agents plus non-pharmacological measures do not achieve adequate glycaemic control.*	In combination with: – Metformin – Acarbose – Thiazolidinedione – Insulin

Fig 4.5

- When hyperglycaemia is severe and there is little improvement with sulphonylurea therapy, it is likely that beta-cell failure is substantial, and insulin should be instituted. When switching from sulphonylurea monotherapy to insulin it may be convenient to continue with low dose sulphonylurea therapy. For example, long-acting bedtime insulin provides a basal exogenous insulin supplement while daytime sulphonylurea therapy can facilitate small endogenous insulin surges into the portal circulation during meal digestion. Meglitinides can be used in a similar manner.

Sulphonylureas: precautions, interactions, contraindications

Precautions
To minimise risk of hypoglycaemia:

- Ensure patient knows how to recognise/respond to symptoms of hypoglycaemia.

- Observe contraindications.

- Select sulphonylurea with pharmacokinetic properties compatible with hepatic/renal status.

Other known medical conditions/therapies:

- Especial caution with longer-acting agents – elderly.

- Potential drug interactions.

- Avoid erratic eating habits *(meglitinides may be more appropriate insulin-releasers in these cases)*.

Drug interactions
Several drugs can either potentiate or reduce hypoglycaemic effect of sulphonylureas (Fig 4.7).

Combination with another glucose-lowering drug class will increase the hypoglycaemic effect.

ACE inhibitors and angiotensin II receptor antagonists may possibly exert a small blood glucose-lowering effect.

Contraindications
Known hypersensitivity
Sensitivity reactions are rare and usually remit promptly on drug's withdrawal.

Type 1 diabetes or previous ketosis
(where there is no endogenous beta-cell function).

Porphyria
(sulphonylureas can acutely aggravate porphyria).

Not recommended in pregnancy or breast-feeding
(substitute insulin).

Fig 4.6

Sites of interaction for drugs potentially *enhancing* the *glucose-lowering effect* of sulphonylureas

Effect on sulphonylurea protein-binding, metabolism and elimination

Displacement from plasma proteins
Sulphonamides
Salicylates (high dose)
Warfarin
Fibrates
Phenylbutazone

Decreased hepatic metabolism
Warfarin
Monoamine oxidase inhibitors
Chloramphenicol
Phenylbutazone and other NSAIDS*
Some antifungals e.g. miconazole

Non-steroidal anti-inflammatory drugs

Decreased renal elimination
Salicylates (high dose)
Probenecid
Allopurinol

Other hypoglycaemic actions

Intrinsic insulin-releasing activity
Salicylates (high dose)
Monoamine oxidase inhibitors
Some quinolone antibacterials

Decreased hepatic gluconeogenesis
Alcohol (excess)

Mask symptoms of hypoglycaemia and reduce counter-regulation
Beta-adrenergic blockers

Fig 4.7

| | | | **Sulphonyureas** |
	Non-proprietary	**Proprietary**	**Tablet strength (mg)**
Tolbutamide	Yes	-	500
Glipizide	Yes	Glibenese, Minodiab	2.5, 5.0 (scored)
Gliquidone	No	Glurenorm	30 (scored)
Gliclazide	Yes	Diamicron	80 (scored)
Gliclazide MR	No	Diamicron MR	30 (scored)
Glimepiride	No	Amaryl	1,2,3,4 (all scored)
Glibenclamide	Yes	Daonil, Semi-Daonil, Euglucon	2.5, 5.0 (scored)
Chlorpropamide*	Yes		100, 250

* Chlorpropamide is less suitable for new patients due to higher incidence of side-effect

Fig 4.8

Sulphonylureas: selection criteria

- Treatment with a sulphonylurea (or any other glucose-lowering drug) should be undertaken as an adjunct to non-pharmacological measures when the latter do not achieve adequate glycaemic control.

- Since all sulphonylureas are metabolised by the liver, and active metabolites of some agents are renally excreted, it is necessary to consider carefully significant liver or renal disease. Sulphonylureas are also highly protein-bound, extending the potential for drug interactions. Choice of sulphonylurea (and decision to exclude sulphonylurea therapy) depends largely on the pharmacokinetic profile that is compatible with the patient's needs, life-style and concurrent medical condition.

- Prescriber experience and preference may also be a factor in this choice.

- **Elderly patients:** *longer-acting agents – chlorpropamide and glibenclamide – are not recommended due to increased risk of hypoglycaemia.*

:art dose ng)	Max daily (mg)	Suggested regimen for max daily dose (mg)	Caution
0	2,000	2,000 mg divided doses with meal	Renal disease
5	20	15 mg o.d., 20 mg divided doses	Renal disease
	180	60 mg o.d.	Hepatic disease
	320	320 mg divided doses	Renal/hepatic disease
	120	120 mg o.d.	Renal/hepatic disease
	6	4 mg o.d. (exceptionally 6 mg o.d.)	Renal/hepatic disease
	15	10 mg o.d. or divided dose (exceptionally 15 mg divided doses)	Renal/hepatic disease, elderly
)	500	500 mg o.d.	Renal disease, elderly

Sulphonylureas: starting therapy

1. Short and short-intermediate-acting agents (tolbutamide, glipizide, gliquidone)

- Usually taken daily before main meals.
- Act mainly against daytime postprandial hyperglycaemia, with less effect on basal nocturnal hyperglycaemia. However, the risk of nocturnal hypoglycaemia should also be reduced.

2. Intermediate-acting (standard gliclazide) and intermediate-long-acting agents (gliclazide MR, glimepiride, glibenclamide)

- Once-daily with breakfast.
- At the upper end of the dosage range may be given in divided doses: a larger proportion of the total daily dosage can be given with breakfast, and a smaller proportion with an early evening meal, to reduce the risk of nocturnal hypoglycaemia.
- The long-acting agent chlorpropamide is usually given once-daily, but is considered less suitable for new therapy, due to a higher incidence of side-effects than other sulphonylureas.

Titration steps

1. Start with a low dose.
   - Monitor glycaemic control by fasting plasma glucose (clinic visits and patient self-monitoring) (see Chapter 2).
2. Increase dosage, usually at intervals of about 2 weeks, until the desired level of glycaemic control is achieved.
   - If symptoms of hypoglycaemia occur:
     - Attempt to acquire confirmation by patient self-monitoring.
     - Reduce dosage one level or adjust diet and exercise schedule accordingly.
   - If hypoglycaemia precludes achieving target control:
     - Consider combination of an acceptable dose of the sulphonylurea with another drug class that does not stimulate insulin release (metformin, thiazolidinedione, acarbose).
     - Alternatively consider switching to a shorter-acting sulphonylurea or a meglitinide, starting at a dosage equivalent to that currently prescribed.
3. Titrate up to the desired level of glycaemic control or the minimum dose with the maximum effect.
   - If an increase in dose does not further improve glycaemic control return to the previous dose (i.e. minimum dose with the maximum therapeutic effect). The maximum therapeutic effect is often achieved well below the maximum recommended dose, as the drug has already produced the maximal insulin secretory response.
4. If a maximally effective dosage of a sulphonylurea does not achieve the desired glycaemic control, or control is achieved but subsequently deteriorates:
   - Consider combination therapy with another drug from another glucose-lowering class that does not stimulate insulin release (e.g. metformin, thiazolidinedione or acarbose).
   - Alternatively, if the hyperglycaemia is marked, consider switching to insulin (see Chapter 8).
5. If transferring from one sulphonylurea to another oral agent (e.g. to a shorter-acting drug due to hypoglycaemia) then start the new therapy at a slightly lower dose-equivalent level than the previous therapy and titrate up if required. Allow a day of washout for chlorpropamide.
6. If starting or withdrawing any potentially interacting therapy it is advised to check glycaemic control and adjust the dose of sulphonylurea if required.

Sulphonylureas: efficacy

The glucose-lowering efficacy of sulphonylureas depends upon adequate remaining beta-cell function, since the main action of these drugs is to stimulate insulin secretion. Since the natural history of type 2 diabetes involves a progressive failure of beta-cells, there is a tendency for blood glucose to gradually and continually rise. Uncontrollable deterioration of glycaemic control with a sulphonylurea (sometimes termed 'secondary sulphonylurea failure') may occur in 5 - 10% of patients each year. Hence periodic reassessment may require increase in drug dosage and recourse to combination therapy, and eventually insulin.

Monotherapy:

HbA1c	↓ 1 - 2%
Fasting plasma glucose	↓ 2 - 4 mmol/L
Onset of effect	Rapid, usually evident on first day of treatment
Near-maximal effect of single dose	Usually 2 weeks

Combination therapy:

- A sulphonylurea can be added when monotherapy with another glucose-lowering drug class (not an insulin-releaser) is unable to achieve or maintain the desired glycaemic control.

- Addition of the sulphonylurea as combination therapy will produce an additive blood glucose-lowering effect, the extent can be similar to monotherapy, but in practice it is usually less due to the progressive decline in beta-cell function.

- Early use of combination therapy is recommended when required to ensure a patient achieves and maintains the desired glycaemic target. Oral combination therapy should not be deferred until hyperglycaemia is marked or used as an inadequate alternative to insulin.

Lipid profile

Minimal change by introduction of a sulphonylurea as monotherapy or combination therapy. Minor improvements in lipid values may occur as a consequence of improved glycaemic control.

Sulphonylureas: adverse effects

Hypoglycaemia
mild, moderate or severe
(see Fig 4.11)

Patients should be made aware of the symptoms, how to respond and to minimise risk of hypoglycaemia.

Hypoglycaemia is more frequent:
– With longer-acting sulphonylureas
– With irregular eating habits
– With good control
– In elderly patients

About 20% of patients receiving a sulphonylurea experience one or more episodes of hypoglycaemia each year, most mild or moderate.

About 1% of patients receiving a sulphonylurea suffer an episode of severe hypoglycaemia each year. Severe sulphonylurea-induced hypoglycaemia must be treated as a medical emergency. However, mortality from sulphonylurea-induced hypoglycaemia is rare (about 0.02 per 1,000 patient years of treatment).

Weight gain

– Typically 1 - 4 kg
– Stabilises after about 6 months
– Common with initiation of sulphonylurea therapy
  probably due to anabolic effect of increased insulin concentrations and reduced loss of glucose in urine.

Sensitivity reactions

Rash (mild) – usually resolves on drug withdrawal.

Photosensitivity, erythema multiforme (rare).

Cholestatic jaundice, hepatitis.

Blood dyscrasias.

Chlorpropamide – Facial flushing with alcohol (Disulfiram effect).
　　　　　　　　– Antidiuretic and hyponatraemic effect (SIADH).

Glibenclamide – May have a mild diuretic effect.

Fig 4.9

Additional point

1. Potential cardiovascular effects due to interactions with SUR2A/B on cardiac and smooth muscle are potentially possible for second generation sulphonylureas with substituted benzamido moiety (glibenclamide, glipizide, glimepiride). Although this could affect vascular adaptations to ischaemia, normal therapeutic use of sulphonylureas does not appear to compromise cardiovascular mortality.

Drugs that can reduce the glucose-lowering effect of sulphonylureas	
Drug	**Site of action**
Diazoxide	Open K^+- ATP channels
Octreotide	Decrease insulin secretion
Glucocorticoids	Antagonise insulin secretion
Nifedipine	Inihibit intracellular calcium flux which in turn inhibits insulin secretion
Loop and thiazide diuretics	Various
Antipsychotic phenothiazines	

Fig 4.10

Categories of hypoglycaemia

	Symptoms	Intervention
Mild	Hunger, sweating, palpitations, tremor	Take glucose-rich sweets, drink or food
Moderate	Cognitive dysfunction, dizziness, atypical behaviour, drowsiness, uncoordinated, speech difficulty	Take glucose-rich sweet or drink and seek assistance
Severe	Reduced consciousness, malaise, headache, nausea, convulsions, coma	Third-party intervention required and/or medical intervention

Fig 4.11

Treatment of sulphonylurea-induced severe hypoglycaemia

1. Exclude alcohol intoxication and acute cerebrovascular event.

2. Administer glucose orally (if conscious) or i.v. (if unconscious).

   – *Administration of glucose should be prolonged to avoid relapse, since longer-acting sulphonylureas can stimulate insulin secretion for >24 h.*

   – *Glucose administration will also accentuate insulin secretion in patients with substantial beta-cell reserves.*

3. Mannitol or dexamethasone can be given for cerebral oedema.

4. Check for hypokalaemia.

5. Alkaline diuresis can be used to eliminate chlorpropamide.

Additional points

• *Glucagon must not be used for sulphonylurea-induced hypoglycaemia, as glucagon is a potent insulin-releaser.*

• *Diazoxide (which opens K^+-ATP channels) will antagonise the effect of excess sulphonylurea.*

• *Adverse cardiovascular effects of diazoxide limit its use.*

Fig 4.12

Sulphonylureas at a glance

Class	Sulphonylureas
Action	Stimulate insulin secretion

Indications*	● *Type 2 diabetes*
	  – Monotherapy
	  – Combination with other antidiabetic agents (metformin, acarbose, thiazolidinediones, insulin) except another insulin-releasing agent

Choice	Select sulphonylurea with duration of action and pharmacokinetic properties that are compatible with patient
Treatment	Start with low dose at breakfast Titrate slowly, and monitor blood glucose Educate patient to recognise, respond to, and prevent hypoglycaemia. Maximum effect is likely to be achieved before the maximum permitted dose is reached
Cautions and contraindications	Use cautiously in patients with hepatic or renal disease (see pharmacokinetics) Avoid patients with porphyria
Efficacy	HbA1c $\downarrow 1$ - 2% FPG and postprandial glycaemia $\downarrow 2$ - 4 mmol/L
Adverse effects	Risk of hypoglycaemia, especially with longer-acting agents Occasionally sensitivity reactions and minor effects on renal sodium and water excretion Chlorpropamide can cause alcohol-induced facial flush
Precautions	Patient education about hypoglycaemia and weight gain Potential drug interactions, e.g. with salicylates, sulphonamides and warfarin

* Indication assumes inadequate glycaemic control with non-pharmacological measures (and existing pharmacological therapy for combination use)

5 MEGLITINIDES

Historical background

1998   Repaglinide introduced.

2001   Nateglinide introduced.

Meglitinides, also known as *prandial insulin-releasers,* are structurally related to the benzamido region of glibenclamide. There are two meglitinides used in clinical practice: **repaglinide** is a benzoic acid derivative, while **nateglinide** is an amino acid derivative of D-phenylalanine. Both are rapidly-acting and short-acting insulin-releasers.

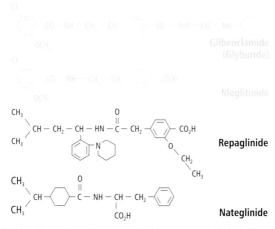

Fig 5.1 Structures of repaglinide and nateglinide showing their similarities to meglitinide and the benzamido region of glibenclamide

The blood glucose-lowering efficacy of meglitinides, like sulphonylureas, requires adequate remaining beta-cell function to allow stimulation of insulin secretion. Meglitinides act directly on pancreatic beta-cells, but with a faster onset and shorter duration of action than sulphonylureas. Taken immediately before a meal, a meglitinide will increase insulin secretion to coincide with the approximate duration of meal digestion. Thus meglitinides are used to increase prandial insulin secretion and will mainly lower postprandial hyperglycaemia.

Meglitinides: pharmacokinetics

Both repaglinide and nateglinide are rapidly absorbed achieving a
maximum plasma concentration within 1 h. Plasma concentrations
of both repaglinide and nateglinide peak and decline rapidly,
approximately in concert with their short duration of action,
whereas drug metabolism and elimination take longer.

Meglitinides: pharmacokinetics		
	Repaglinide	**Nateglinide**
Bioavailability	50 - 60%	~70%
Time to peak plasma concentration	<1 h	<1 h
Plasma protein-binding	>98%	>97%
Metabolism main metabolic pathway	Liver (100%) CYP3A4	Liver (>85%) CYP2C9 and CYP3A4
Metabolites	Dicarboxylic-Amine Glucuronide	Hydroxy-Others
Activity of metabolites	Inactive	One minor metabolite is active
Elimination t½	~1.5 h	~1.5 h
Elimination	Bile ~90%	Urine ~80%

Fig 5.2

Meglitinides: mode of action

- The rapid stimulation of insulin secretion by meglitinides at the beginning of meal digestion mimics the acute (first) phase of insulin secretion that normally occurs at the beginning of meal digestion. This acute phase of insulin secretion is lost in type 2 diabetes.

- The acute phase insulin response provides a surge of insulin to the liver to suppress hepatic glucose production. Inadequate suppression of hepatic glucose production in type 2 diabetes appears to make a substantial contribution to the exaggerated postprandial hyperglycaemia. Accordingly, the acute stimulation of insulin secretion by meglitinides taken with meals predominantly reduces postprandial hyperglycaemia.

Meglitinides: mode of action	
Pancreatic *(main effect)*	1. Stimulate insulin secretion.
	2. Initiate insulin secretion at low glucose concentrations.
	3. Enhance glucose-stimulated insulin release.
	Dependent on functional pancreatic beta-cells in the islets of Langerhans. *Drug binds to the benzamido site on sulphonylurea receptor (SUR-1) of beta-cells.* **The benzamido site is distinct from the sulphonylurea binding site.**
Mechanism	→ *Closure of K^+- ATP channels reduces potassium efflux.*
	→ *Local intracellular retention of potassium causes membrane depolarisation which opens voltage-dependent calcium influx channels.*
	→ *Rise in intracellular free calcium concentration activates calcium-dependent proteins with release (exocytosis) of insulin granules.*

Fig 5.3

Mechanism of insulin release stimulated by meglitinides

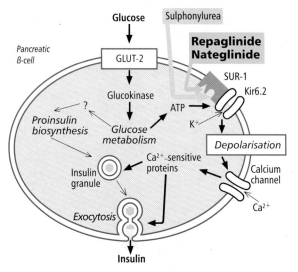

Fig 5.4

Therapeutic distinction between meglitinides and sulphonylureas

1. More rapid onset and shorter duration of insulin secretion.
2. Fast absorption and metabolism.
3. Relatively short duration of binding and closure of K^+-ATP channels.

   – Hence a meglitinide can be taken with the meal and stimulate insulin release for the period of meal digestion.

   – The short duration of effect is less likely to cause interprandial hypoglycaemia.

Fig 5.5

Postprandial profiles following standard meal test

(1) Mean glucose

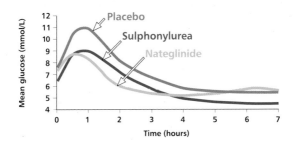

(2) Mean incremental glucose

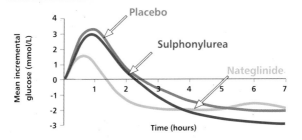

(3) Insulin secretion profile

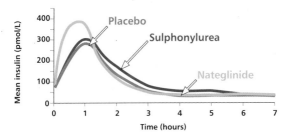

Values at time 0 obtained prior to study medication and standard breakfast in a person with type 2 diabetes.

Fig 5.6 **Nateglinide and repaglinide produce a faster plasma insulin response and a lower postprandial glucose excursion to a standard meal than a sulphonylurea or placebo**

Meglitinides: indications

- Especially useful for postprandial (rather than basal) hyperglycaemia.
- Preference for a meglitinide instead of a sulphonylurea:
  - With irregular, erratic and unpredictable life-style and eating habits, including missed meals.
  - Interprandial hypoglycaemia, for example during sulphonylurea therapy.
- Elderly – observe contraindications.
- Renal insufficiency – dose adjustment with nateglinide may be required in patients on dialysis.

Meglitinides: indications		
Type 2 diabetes non-obese or obese	**Repaglinide** First-line monotherapy *when there is inadequate glycaemic control by non-pharmacological measures.*	
	Second-line drug therapy *when monotherapy with other agents plus non-pharmacological measures do not achieve adequate glycaemic control.*	In combination with: – Metformin – Acarbose – Insulin – Thiazolidinedione
	Nateglinide Second-line drug therapy *when monotherapy with metformin plus non-pharmacological measures do not achieve adequate glycaemic control.*	In combination with: – Metformin
		Present permitted indication for nateglinide is somewhat restrictive.

Fig 5.7

Additional points

1. The same general precautions regarding drug interactions apply as described for sulphonylureas.
2. In practice, little clinically significant interaction with meglitinides has been reported.

Meglitinides: precautions, interactions, contraindications

Precautions

To minimise risk of hypoglycaemia:
- Ensure patient knows how to recognise /respond to symptoms of hypoglycaemia.
- Observe contraindications.
- Risk of hypoglycaemia should be minimised by observing contraindications, checking glycaemic control and providing clear advice on the use of flexible mealtime dosing regimen.

Potential drug interactions
Moderate hepatic impairment

Drug interactions

Increasing the risk of hypoglycaemia

Combination with another glucose-lowering drug,
ACE inhibitor or angiotensin II blocker

Increasing metabolism and reducing effectiveness
- Inducers of P450 CYP3A4, and CYP2C9 may increase metabolism of meglitinides
- Use of drug with inherent hyperglycaemic effects or an oral contraceptive may necessitate adjustments to therapy

Rifampicin
Barbiturates
Carbamazepine

Increasing meglitinide activity
- Inhibition of hepatic CYP3A4 increases potential risk of increasing meglitinide activity
- Inhibition of CYP2C9 could affect nateglinide
- Highly protein-bound drugs may displace meglitinides

Erythromycin and some antifungal agents

Some non-steroidal anti-inflammatory agents,
salicylates,
sulphonamides,
warfarin monoamine oxidase inhibitors

Contraindications

Type 1 diabetes or previous ketosis
Severe hepatic impairment
Known hypersensitivity to these drugs
Not recommended in pregnancy, breast-feeding or children as safety has not been established.

Fig 5.8

Meglitinides: starting therapy

- Use of a meglitinide assumes use as an adjunct to non-pharmacological measures when these measures do not achieve adequate glycaemic control in type 2 diabetes.
- Repaglinide can be used as monotherapy or combination therapy.
- Nateglinide is restricted to combination therapy with metformin.

Patients with mainly postprandial (rather than basal) hyperglycaemia, and those with irregular life-styles are most suitable. Follow the same general principles as starting a sulphonylurea (see Fig 4.8).

Titration steps

1. Start with a low dose e.g. 0.5 mg repaglinide or 60 mg nateglinide (plus metformin) with two or three main meals daily.
2. Take up to 30 minutes before or during the meal; preferably take when about to begin the meal.
3. Monitor glycaemic control by patient self-monitoring at 1 h or 2 h after beginning a meal. Also check fasting glucose values.
4. Increase dosage at intervals of about 1 - 2 weeks until the desired level of glycaemic control is achieved.
5. If symptoms of hypoglycaemia occur or a titration step produces no further improvement in glycaemic control, revert to the previous dosage level.
6. Maximum recommended dosage is:
   - Repaglinide 4 mg with any one meal, up to 16 mg daily.
   - Nateglinide 180 mg with any one meal, up to 540 mg daily.
7. If desired target for glycaemic control is not achieved:
   - Consider oral combination with another class of antidiabetic agent if taking repaglinide as monotherapy.
   - Consider switching to insulin if already taking a combination of oral antidiabetic drugs.

Selecting a meglitinide *(prandial insulin-releaser)*

	Repaglinide	Nateglinide
Proprietary name *No generic agent available*	NovoNorm	Starlix
Tablet strengths (mg)	0.5, 1, 2	60, 120, 180
Monotherapy indication available	Yes	No
Start dose (mg)	0.5	60
Suggested max daily (mg)	16 (4 mg with each meal)	540 (180 mg with each meal)
Caution	Hepatic disease	Hepatic disease

Fig 5.9

Meglitinides: efficacy

- During chronic therapy the effect of meglitinides is usually evident on the first day of treatment and will be near maximal by about one week.

- Postprandial glucose concentrations are often reduced ~one-third.
  - *Appropriate postprandial glucose target for self-monitoring is <8 mmol/L at 1 - 2 hours after a meal.*

- Although the predominant effect of meglitinides is to reduce postprandial hyperglycaemia, there is some 'carry-over' effect to improve basal glycaemia, hence the reduction in fasting plasma glucose.

Monotherapy (with repaglinide):

HbA1c	↓1 - 2%
Fasting plasma glucose	↓1 - 3 mmol/L

Combination therapy:

- Slightly lesser effect, probably because the natural history of the disease will be more advanced, and beta-cell function will be more severely compromised.

- Additive decreases:
  - HbA1c ↓0.5 - 1.5%
  - Fasting plasma glucose ↓0.7 - 2 mmol/L

Lipid profile

No significant changes have been reported.

Meglitinides: adverse effects	
Hypoglycaemia	Patients should be made aware of the symptoms, how to respond and to minimise risk of hypoglycaemia.
	Since meglitinides are short-acting insulin secretagogues they are less likely to cause severe hypoglycaemia than sulphonylureas.
	Recurrent hypoglycaemia with meglitinides may require a dose change. Check that medication is taken at an appropriate time relative to the start and composition of the meal.
	Combination with metformin or a thiazolidinedione may help to reduce the risk of severe hypoglycaemia in patients with good glycaemic control.
Weight gain (Repaglinide only)	– Generally small, 1 - 3 kg – Stabilises in 3 - 6 months
Sensitivity reactions	Rash (mild), itching urticaria, usually transient – resolves on drug withdrawal
	Hypersensitivity (rare)
	Raised LFTs (nateglinide) – transient

Fig 5.10

Additional point

1. *Cardiovascular effects:* Meglitinides possess the potential to bind to the benzamido site of SUR2A/B on K^+-ATP channels of cardiac and smooth muscle. However, there is no evidence of any clinically significant cardiovascular interactions.

Meglitinides at a glance

Class	Meglitinides (prandial insulin-releasers)
Action	Short-acting stimulators of insulin secretion
Indications[*]	• *Type 2 diabetes* *Repaglinide* – Monotherapy – Combination with other antidiabetic agents except another insulin-releasing agent *Nateglinide* – Combination with metformin
Choice	Faster-acting and shorter-acting than sulphonylureas Opportunity for flexible mealtime administration
Treatment	Start with low dose with each main meal Titrate at intervals of 1 - 2 weeks and monitor blood glucose Explain importance of taking with meals and dealing with hypoglycaemia
Cautions and contraindications	Avoid patients with severe liver disease
Efficacy	*Monotherapy with repaglinide* HbA1c $\downarrow$1 - 2% FPG $\downarrow$1 - 3 mmol/L Postprandial glycaemia $\downarrow$1 - 4 mmol/L *Combination: additional effect* HbA1c $\downarrow$0.5 - 1.5% FPG $\downarrow$1 - 3 mmol/L Postprandial glycaemia $\downarrow$1 - 3 mmol/L
Adverse effects	Risk of hypoglycaemia Rarely sensitivity reactions
Precautions	Potential drug interactions with protein-bound drugs e.g. salicylates, sulphonamides, warfarin and agents affecting CYP3A4 and CYP2C9 (nateglinide)

[*] Indication assumes inadequate glycaemic control with non-pharmacological measures (and existing pharmacological therapy for combination use)

6 BIGUANIDES

Historical background

'Medieval times'	*Galega officinalis* (Goat's rue or French Lillac) used as traditional treatment for diabetes in Europe.
1850	*Galega officinalis* found to be rich in guanidine.
1918	Guanidine shown to lower blood glucose.
1920	Various biguanides and diguanides synthesised and shown to lower blood glucose.
Post 1920s	Insulin era: biguanides forgotten.
1957	Metformin and phenformin described.
1958	Buformin described.
1960s	Biguanides – metformin, phenformin and buformin – introduced widely, especially phenformin.
Late 1970s	Phenformin and buformin withdrawn from most countries due to a high incidence of associated lactic acidosis.
1995	Metformin introduced into USA.
1998	United Kingdom Prospective Diabetes Study (UKPDS): Metformin improves microvascular and macrovascular outcomes.
2001	Diabetes Prevention Program (DPP): Metformin reduces progression of IGT to type 2 diabetes.

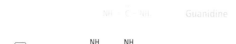

Fig 6.1 Structures of guanidine, phenformin, buformin and metformin

- Metformin is now used widely in clinical practice and is the preferred initial oral therapy for overweight and obese individuals with type 2 diabetes.
- Metformin counters insulin resistance by increasing insulin sensitivity and by some actions that are not directly insulin-dependent. It reduces mainly basal hyperglycaemia, but does not cause overt hypoglycaemia, does not stimulate insulin secretion and does not cause weight gain. Additional effects on the lipid profile and thrombotic factors may also reduce cardiovascular risk. Metformin can cause unwelcome gastrointestinal responses in some patients (lessened with prolonged release formulation), and carries a risk of lactic acidosis if wrongly prescribed.

Metformin: pharmacokinetics

- Metformin (hydrochloride) is rapidly absorbed (1 - 3 h) mainly from the upper small intestine (4 - 8 h for prolonged release formulation).
- Metformin quickly distributes to most tissues at concentrations similar to those in peripheral plasma (maximally 1 - 2 μg/mL, about 10^{-5} M). Higher concentrations are found in the liver, kidney and salivary glands, and high concentrations are retained in the intestinal wall, which serves as a reservoir of the drug.
- Over 90% of a single dose is eliminated in twenty-four hours, partly by glomerular filtration and partly by renal tubular secretion.

Metformin: pharmacokinetics	
Bioavailability	50 - 60%, declining slightly with high dosages
Peak plasma concentration	1 - 2 μg/ml
Time to peak plasma concentration	1 - 3 h (4 - 8 h for prolonged release formulation)
Plasma protein-binding	Negligible
Metabolism	Not metabolised
Elimination t½	~6 h
Elimination	Urine ~100%
Duration of action	6 - 16 h (up to 24 h for prolonged release formulation)

Fig 6.2

Metformin: mode of action

Metformin is an *antihyperglycaemic* (rather than a hypoglycaemic) drug and (like acarbose and thiazolidinediones) does not lower plasma glucose concentrations below the normal range and therefore does not cause hypoglycaemia.

The antihyperglycaemic efficacy of metformin requires the presence of insulin but metformin does not raise basal insulin concentrations. Some effects of metformin involve increased insulin action (insulin 'sensitising' effect) and other effects are independent of insulin action. Overall, the effects of metformin are extrapancreatic and serve to combat insulin resistance.

Antihyperglycaemic actions of metformin

1. Suppression of hepatic glucose production.
2. Increased insulin-mediated muscle glucose uptake.
3. Decreased fatty acid oxidation.
4. Increased intestinal glucose utilisation.

Fig 6.3

Metformin: mode of action

Hepatic effects	Lowers fasting hyperglycaemia by: • Reduced hepatic gluconeogenesis (main effect) • Reduced glycogenolysis (lesser effect) *These effects mostly reflect potentiation of hepatic insulin action and a reduced hepatic effect of glucagon.* • Reduced lactate extraction • Impede the activity of hepatic glucose-6-phosphatase
Skeletal muscle effects	• *Enhances insulin-mediated glucose uptake and utilisation by up to approximately 20%.* *This effect is associated with increased translocation of insulin-sensitive glucose transporters into the cell membrane.*
Insulin-independent effects	• *Suppression of fatty acid oxidation and decrease in hypertriglyceridaemia will reduce the supply of energy for gluconeogenesis and improve the glucose-fatty acid (Randle) cycle.* • *Increased glucose turnover, due to increased anaerobic glucose utilisation by the intestine. This action is likely to benefit the weight-stabilising or weight-reducing effect of metformin as well as glucose-lowering.*

Fig 6.4

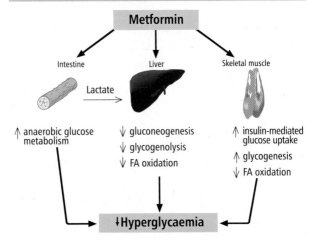

The antihyperglycaemic actions of metformin

Metformin

Intestine

Liver

Skeletal muscle

Lactate →

↑ anaerobic glucose metabolism

↓ gluconeogenesis
↓ glycogenolysis
↓ FA oxidation

↑ insulin-mediated glucose uptake
↑ glycogenesis
↓ FA oxidation

↓ **Hyperglycaemia**

Fig 6.5

Metformin: effects on the metabolic syndrome

- Consistent with its actions to counter insulin resistance, and additional to its antihyperglycaemic effects, metformin has been reported to ameliorate several cardiovascular risk factors of the metabolic syndrome (*insulin resistance syndrome*).

- Such effects could contribute to reduced macrovascular complications and increased survival observed in overweight type 2 diabetic patients who received metformin as initial glucose-lowering drug therapy in the United Kingdom Prospective Diabetes Study (UKPDS).

Effects of metformin on the metabolic syndrome

Insulin resistance — Counters insulin resistance, e.g. improves insulin action in type 2 diabetes.

Hyperinsulinaemia — Reduces fasting hyperinsulinaemia and proinsulin.

Abdominal obesity — Usually stabilises body weight; reduces weight gain and facilitates weight loss.

Hyperglycaemia — Improves glycaemic control in type 2 diabetes and reduces progression of impaired glucose tolerance (IGT) to type 2 diabetes.

Dyslipidaemia — Modest improvements to lipid profile often seen in dyslipidaemic patients, e.g. ↓VLDL-TG, ↓LDL-C, ↑HDL-C.

Hypertension — No significant effect on blood pressure in most studies.

Pro-coagulant state — Some antithrombotic effects, e.g. ↓PAI-1, ↓fibrinogen, ↓platelet aggregation.

Atherosclerosis — Pre-clinical studies showing antiatherogenic effects; no equivalent clinical studies.

VLDL – *very low density lipoprotein*
TG – *triglyceride*
LDL-C – *low density lipoprotein cholesterol*
HDL-C – *high density lipoprotein cholesterol*
PAI-1 – *plasminogen activator inhibitor-1*

Fig 6.6

Metformin: indications

Metformin is usually the preferred initial oral drug therapy in overweight and obese patients because it does not cause weight gain and can assist in modest weight loss.

Metformin: indications		
Type 2 diabetes *non-obese or obese*	First-line monotherapy *when there is inadequate glycaemic control by non-pharmacological measures.*	
	Second-line drug therapy *when monotherapy with other agents plus non-pharmacological measures do not achieve adequate glycaemic control.*	In combination with: – Sulphonylurea – Acarbose – Repaglinide – Thiazolidinedione – Insulin

Fig 6.7

- Metformin reduced cardiovascular morbidity and mortality in patients initially treated with this drug in the United Kingdom Prospective Diabetes Study (UKPDS).

- Use of metformin requires some circulating insulin present. This implies adequate remaining beta-cell function (unless the patient is already receiving insulin). When hyperglycaemia is severe and there is little improvement with metformin monotherapy or oral combination therapy, it is likely that there is marked beta-cell failure, and insulin should be considered. If switching to insulin from an oral regimen involving metformin (monotherapy or combination) it may be convenient to continue some level of metformin therapy, *e.g. long-acting bedtime insulin provides a basal exogenous insulin supplement while daytime metformin therapy can improve insulin action, reduce insulin dosage and facilitate glycaemic control without additional short-acting daytime insulin injections.*

Elderly and young (<18 years of age) patients

Use with caution provided the patient has adequate renal function and preferably the dose is not titrated to the maximum.

Use in type 1 diabetes

While metformin is not effective as a primary treatment in type 1 diabetes, it can be used to reduce insulin dosage and improve control in insulin-treated patients.

Metformin: starting therapy

- Metformin is generally regarded as the initial oral agent of choice for overweight and obese type 2 patients.

- Treatment with metformin, like other oral antidiabetic agents, should be undertaken as an adjunct to non-pharmacological measures when these measures do not achieve adequate glycaemic control.

- Ensure no contraindication (see Fig 6.8).

Titration steps

1. Start with a low dose, e.g. one 500 mg or 850 mg tablet at breakfast or other main meal.

2. Monitor glycaemic control by fasting plasma glucose at clinic visits and patient self-monitoring (see Chapter 2).

3. Increase the dose every 1 - 2 weeks by one tablet at a time, always taking the drug with a main meal. For example, increase to one tablet with each of two or three main meals, and then in divided daily doses with the main meals.

4. Continue increasing the dosage until the desired level of glycaemic control is achieved.

5. If a titration step does not improve glycaemic control return to the previous dosage level (i.e. the minimum dose with the maximum therapeutic effect). The maximum therapeutic effect is often achieved by 1,750 - 2,550 mg daily, i.e. below the maximum recommended dose of 3,000 mg daily.

If gastrointestinal symptoms occur:

- Revert to the previous dosage level and re-titrate if the symptoms remit or try prolonged release formulation of metformin.

- If the symptoms are very mild, remain at that dosage level for 2 - 4 weeks to see if they remit.

- If the symptoms are severe and do not remit, consider an alternative treatment (symptoms invariably remit quickly when metformin is discontinued).

Slow titration and taking metformin with the main meals should minimalise gastrointestinal symptoms.

*If a maximally effective dose of metformin does **not** achieve the desired glycaemic control, or control is achieved but subsequently deteriorates:*

- Consider combination therapy by adding another oral glucose-lowering drug (sulphonylurea, meglitinide, acarbose or thiazolidinedione). Current guidelines suggest trying a metformin-sulphonylurea combination before a metformin-thiazolidinedione combination.

- Alternatively, if the hyperglycaemia is marked, consider switching to insulin (see Chapter 8).

If symptoms of hypoglycaemia occur, these are only likely to be severe if metformin is being used in combination with another antidiabetic agent, usually an insulin-releaser or insulin itself:

- Attempt to acquire confirmation by patient self-monitoring of blood glucose.

- Reduce dosage level of one agent (usually the insulin-releaser or insulin rather than metformin) and adjust diet and exercise schedule accordingly.

If hypoglycaemia precludes achieving target glycaemic control with metformin combined with an insulin-releaser:

- Consider combination of metformin with a shorter-acting insulin-releaser, or a thiazolidinedione or acarbose.

If transferring from a combination of metformin-sulphonylurea or metformin-meglitinide to metformin-thiazolidinedione, the licencing restrictions preclude triple therapy and, in principle, require the insulin-releaser to be stopped as the thiazolidinedione is started. Since a thiazolidinedione will often take 1 - 3 months to reach full efficacy, this can lead to a loss of glycaemic control. Therefore, a period of triple therapy may be helpful.

Prescribers must take responsibility to explain the situation and receive the informed agreement of the patient if electing to recommend to titrate down the insulin-releaser in concert with the introduction and up-titration of the thiazolidinedione. This must be undertaken with care, e.g. increased potential for hypoglycaemia, and the dosages of all agents must be reviewed frequently while monitoring glycaemic control. Despite being outside the licence this manoeuvre has been undertaken carefully to retain glycaemic control.

Metformin: efficacy

Development of the glucose-lowering effect is usually more gradual than with an insulin-releaser, consonent with slower titration (and administration with meals) to minimise initial gastrointestinal responses.

Monotherapy:

HbAlc	↓1 - 2%
Fasting plasma glucose	↓1 - 4 mmol/L
Likely to slightly reduce	Basal insulin concentrations
Likely to slightly improve	Lipid concentrations in dyslipidaemic patients *(decrease VLDL-TG, LDL-C and FFA, increase HDL-C). The magnitude of the lipid effects is about 5 - 15%.*

Unlikely to cause significant hypoglycaemia

Unlikely to cause significant weight gain

- Co-administration of drugs with inherent hyperglycaemic effects (e.g. glucocorticoids) may necessitate an increase in metformin dosage.

- About 20% of patients experience gastrointestinal symptoms with metformin, even when titrated appropriately. While these mostly remit by further slowing the titration process, about 5% of patients do not tolerate metformin. Prolonged release formulation of metformin can reduce gastrointestinal symptoms.

- Only a small minority of type 2 patients titrated up on metformin fail to show a clinically significant response. Such patients are likely to be severely insulinopenic and advanced in the natural history of the disease.

- The progressive nature of type 2 diabetes, which is associated with a continual deterioration in glycaemic control, is likely to:
  – Require periodic adjustment of dosage and eventual recourse to combination therapy.

  About 5 - 10% of patients per year who are treated with metformin will experience a marked deterioration in glycaemic control, as seen with other oral glucose-lowering drugs. This is due mainly to the continued loss of beta-cell function in type 2 diabetes.

Combination therapy:

- Metformin can be added when monotherapy with another oral agent or insulin does not provide the desired glycaemic control or insulin dosage is excessive.

- Metformin combination therapy will produce an additive blood glucose-lowering effect. The extent of this effect can be similar to monotherapy, but in practice it is usually less because of the natural history of the disease and beta-cell function is further reduced.

- Early use of combination therapy is recommended to ensure the desired glycaemic target is maintained.

   The UKPDS found that after three years about 50% of patients on monotherapy with metformin or a sulphonylurea will experience inadequate glycaemic control (e.g. HbA1c >7%) rising to about 75% of patients after nine years. Thus the majority of patients are likely to require combination therapy to retain glycaemic control, and this should be implemented without delay when glycaemic control becomes unsatisfactory despite appropriate titration of the monotherapy.

- Severe and rapidly rising hyperglycaemia usually signals the need to switch to insulin.

Metformin: precautions, interactions, contraindications

Precautions
- Observe all contraindications.
- Slow titration.
- Administer with main meals to reduce gastrointestinal symptoms.
- Monitor   Serum creatinine (e.g. annually), or more frequently if deterioration is suspected.

                       Haemoglobin (e.g. annually).

- Make routine checks to ensure contraindications have not developed.
- Special vigilance in the young and elderly.
  Creatinine clearance test may be advisable for patients in the 8th decade.

Ovulation can restart in anovulatory polycystic ovary syndrome (PCOS).
Contraceptive awareness should be ensured in pre-menopausal PCOS patients.

Withhold metformin   During use of intravenous radiographic contrast media
           (until normal urine flow is resumed)
           During major surgery
           (temporary switch to insulin is preferred)

Risk of hyperlactataemia and lactic acidosis
1. Reduced renal function.
   As metformin is eliminated in the urine reduced renal function may produce accumulation of excess metformin.
2. Hypoperfusion or tissue hypoxia are exclusions (list below).

Drug interactions

Cimetidine	*Metformin levels are increased due to the same renal tubular transporters.*
Cationic drugs	*Theoretically, interactions could occur, but these have not been observed in practice.*
Furosemide	*Minor pharmacokinetic interactions occur.*
Nifedipine	*Minor pharmacokinetic interactions occur.*

Contraindications
Renal disease/dysfunction.
Abnormal creatinine clearance test or raised serum creatinine >130 µmol/L.
Any condition predisposing to hypoperfusion and tissue hypoxia.
Cardiac insufficiency such as congestive heart disease or recent myocardial infarction
Severe respiratory insufficiency
Acute shock
Septicaemia or severe infection
History of lactic acid or other metabolic acidosis including diabetic ketoacidosis.
Significant liver disease.
Alcohol abuse.
Known hypersensitivity to metformin.
Pregnancy and breast-feeding.

Fig 6.8

Metformin: adverse effects

Lactic acidosis

Rare (potential serious concern with metformin).

Presentation is variable and non-specific, and treatment must be immediate, before a laboratory determination of plasma metformin to establish whether an accumulation of the drug has occurred (see Fig 6.8).

– Incidence is about 0.03 per 1,000 patient years with a 50% mortality.
– Usually occurs because a contraindication has been overlooked, e.g. deterioration of renal function or congestive heart failure.
– Not all cases of lactic acidosis in patients receiving metformin will be related to the drug therapy. The incidence rate of lactic acidosis in type 2 diabetes in patients not receiving metformin is not established.

Gastrointestinal side-effects

– Nausea
– Metallic taste
– Non-specific abdominal discomfort
– Diarrhoea

Effects can be minimised by taking metformin with meals or taking prolonged release formulation.

Symptoms may remit spontaneously with time but usually require a reduction in dosage (especially diarrhoea) or discontinuation of drug if the effects are severe or unresponsive to dosage reduction.
– Occur in about 20% starting metformin.
– 5% of patients do not tolerate the drug.

Reduced absorption of vitamin B$_{12}$ and folate

Rarely associated with anaemia.

Resolves quickly if metformin withdrawn.

Annual measurement of haemoglobin (or vitamin B$_{12}$) recommended.

– The condition appears to be due to interference of metformin with the intrinsic factor-B$_{12}$ complex and may respond to more dietary calcium.
– Affects <10% of patients (often related to poor diet).

Hypoglycaemia

May be clinically significant if metformin given with insulin-releasing agent or with insulin.

Fig 6.9

Presenting features and treatment of lactic acidosis

1. **Presenting signs and symptoms:**

   Often non-specific   Malaise
   Myalgia   Hyperventilation
   Hypothermia   Hypotension
   Generalised abdominal discomfort Somnolence

2. **Diagnosis:**

   Arterial lactate >5 mmol/L

   Arterial pH <7.25

   Anion gap $[Na^+]-[Cl^- + HCO_3^-]$ >15 mmol/L

   Lactic acidosis associated with metformin accumulation
   – *(plasma metformin >5 μg/mL)*

   Suspect lactic acidosis if a diabetic patient presents with metabolic acidosis without ketonuria or ketonaemia and not significantly dehydrated.

3. **Treatment:**

   Hospital emergency-supportive measures.

   Stop metformin;

   if metformin level raised
   – *prompt haemodialysis to remove metformin and correct the acidosis.*

Fig 6.10

Metformin at a glance

Class	Biguanide
Action	Counters insulin resistance

Indications[*]	● *Type 2 diabetes*
	  – Monotherapy
	  – Combination with other antidiabetic agents
	    (sulphonylureas, meglitinides, acarbose,
	    thiazolidinediones, insulin)

Choice	Usually preferred for overweight and obese patients
Treatment	Start with low dose, e.g. 500 mg, titrate slowly, always take with meals – Maximum recommended dose 2 - 2.55 g/day – Maximum permitted dose 3 g/ day
Cautions and contraindications	Renal disease or dysfunction (e.g. creatinine >130 μmol/L) Any condition predisposing to hypoperfusion and hypoxia such as: – Cardiac insufficiency, e.g. congestive heart disease – Severe respiratory insufficiency – Acute shock – Septicaemia or severe infection History of lactic acidosis or other metabolic acidosis Significant liver disease or alcohol abuse Pregnancy and breast-feeding
Efficacy	HbA1c $\downarrow$1 - 2% FPG and postprandial glycaemia $\downarrow$2 - 4 mmol/L Not cause hypoglycaemia as monotherapy Additional effects against metabolic syndrome, e.g: – Not cause weight gain – Can improve lipid profile – Reduced thrombotic factors – Reduced basal hyperinsulinaemia
Adverse effects	Risk of lactic acidosis with a contraindication Gastrointestinal disturbances Reduced absorption of vitamin B_{12} Hypoglycaemia if used in combination with an insulin-releaser or insulin
Precautions	Monitor for contraindications Check serum creatinine and haemoglobin Possible interaction with cimetidine therapy Possible restart of ovulation in PCOS Withhold during use of radiographic contrast media and major surgery

[*] Indication assumes inadequate glycaemic control with non-pharmacological measures (and existing pharmacological therapy for combination use)

Historical background

1982	Ciglitazone, first thiazolidinedione, glucose-lowering effect observed in obese and diabetic animals.
1980-90s	Thiazolidinediones developed for use in treatment of type 2 diabetes.
1997	Troglitazone introduced into clinical practice.
Late 1997	Troglitazone withdrawn due to idiosyncratic hepatotoxicity.
2000	Rosiglitazone and pioglitazone introduced into clinical practice.
2003	Rosiglitazone-metformin combination as a single tablet.

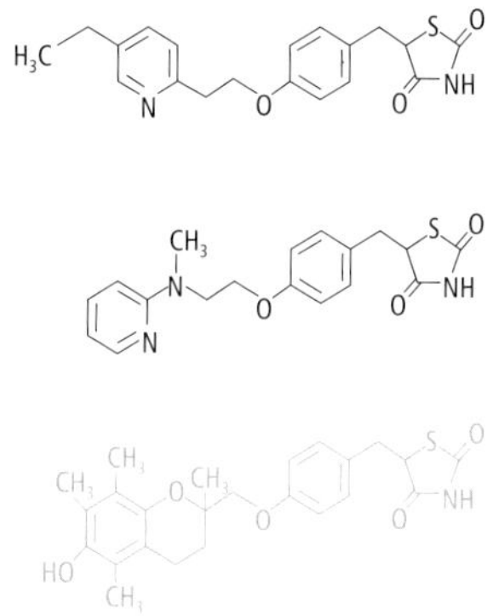

Pioglitazone

Rosiglitazone

Troglitazone

Fig 7.1 Structures of thiazolidinediones

Thiazolidinediones (TZDs), known as 'glitazones', improve insulin action ('*insulin sensitizers*') mainly by activating a nuclear receptor called peroxisome proliferator-activated receptor-gamma (PPARγ). This promotes transcription of several genes that are also responsive to insulin.

A thiazolidine-2,4-dione structure is common to all drugs in the class, with pharmacological and side-effect differences being determined by modifications in the side-chain. Troglitazone, a thiazolidinedione linked to an α-tocopherol (vitamin E) moiety, is strongly lipophilic and may induce liver enzymes. Due to idiosyncratic hepatotoxicity troglitazone was withdrawn from clinical practice.

Thiazolidinediones in current clinical use are rosiglitazone (maleate salt) and pioglitazone (hydrochloride).

Thiazolidinediones: pharmacokinetics

Both rosiglitazone and pioglitazone are rapidly, almost completely absorbed, highly protein-bound and metabolised quickly by the liver.

- Rosiglitazone is almost entirely metabolised to inactive metabolites, two-thirds of which are eliminated in the urine.
- Pioglitazone is metabolised to several active metabolites. The circulating concentrations of the metabolites of pioglitazone are greater than the drug itself, and unmetabolised drug and metabolites are eliminated mainly in the bile.

Rosiglitazone and pioglitazone: pharmacokinetics

	Rosiglitazone	Pioglitazone
Bioavailability	~99%	Almost complete
Time to peak concentration	~1 h	<2 h
Plasma protein-binding	>99%	>99%
Metabolism enzyme pathway	Liver CYP2C8 and CYP2C9	Liver CYP2C8, CYP3A4 and other P450 isoforms
Metabolites	Hydroxy- Demethyl-	Hydroxy- Keto-
Activity of metabolites	Very weak activity (no contribution to therapeutic effect)	Active
Elimination t$\frac{1}{2}$	3 - 4 h (100 - 160 h) (includes metabolites)	3 - 7 h (16 - 24 h) (includes metabolites)
Elimination	Urine ~64%	Bile >60%

Fig 7.2

Thiazolidinediones: mode of action

Thiazolidinediones increase insulin action principally as *agonists of the nuclear peroxisome proliferator-activated receptor-gamma (PPARγ)*. This receptor, which complexes with the retinoid X receptor (RXR), is found mostly in adipose tissue.

Peroxisome proliferator-activated receptor-gamma (PPARγ) receptor/features	
Tissues: Strong expression	Adipose tissue
Weak expression	Skeletal muscle, liver
Genes activated	Lipoprotein lipase (LPL)
	Fatty acid transporter protein (FATP)
	Acyl CoA synthetase
	Malic enzyme
	GLUT 4 (glucose transporter isoform 4)
Biological effects	↑ Adipogenesis
	↑ Fatty acid and glucose uptake
	↑ Lipogenesis
Ligands: Natural	Prostaglandin metabolites
Drugs	***Thiazolidinediones***

Fig 7.3

Stimulation of PPARγ by thiazolidinediones

Stimulation of PPARγ TZDs promotes transcription of genes that are also sensitive to insulin (Fig 7.4). The main enzymes and transporters that are produced (Fig 7.3) increase differentiation of new adipocytes, increase uptake of fatty acids and glucose, increase lipogenesis and decrease the release of fatty acids into the circulation. This decreases blood glucose mainly via the glucose-fatty acid (Randle) cycle (Fig 7.5). Thus increased lipogenesis by adipocytes reduces circulating free fatty acid concentrations. This reduces the availability of fatty acids as an energy source for gluconeogenesis in the liver. The re-balanced Randle cycle also reduces the supply of fatty acids to muscles, which then use more glucose instead.

Other actions of thiazolidinediones

- Other TZD-induced glucose-lowering effects include decreased production of the adipocyte cytokine tumour necrosis factor-alpha (TNFα) which contributes to insulin resistance. PPARγ is modestly expressed by liver and muscle, and TZDs may act directly on these tissues to increase insulin action. Some effects of TZDs may also be independent of PPARγ.

- Since PPARγ is expressed to some extent by a range of tissues (Fig 7.3) it is not unexpected that TZDs will have other effects, but these are not yet clearly defined. PPARγ is expressed by pancreatic beta-cells, with pre-clinical evidence indicating that TZDs can preserve or increase insulin granulation and beta-cell mass.

Thiazolidinedione effects

TZDs act more strongly to stimulate glucose uptake and utilisation by *muscle* than suppression of glucose production by liver. In contrast, metformin appears to suppress hepatic glucose production more strongly than it stimulates muscle glucose utilisation. Hence the effects of the two classes of agents are complementary.

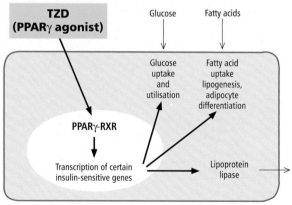

Mechanism of action of a thiazolidinedione (TZD) to activate PPARγ in white adipose tissue

TZD = thiazolidinedione
PPARγ-RXR = peroxisome proliferator-activated receptor-gamma complexed with retinoid X receptor

Fig 7.4

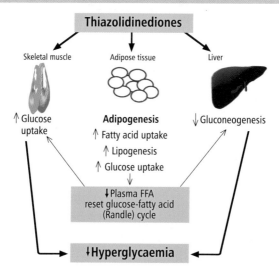

Mechanisms by which thiazolidinediones (PPARγ agonists) reduce hyperglycaemia

Thiazolidinediones

Skeletal muscle ↑ Glucose uptake

Adipose tissue

Adipogenesis
↑ Fatty acid uptake
↑ Lipogenesis
↑ Glucose uptake
↓
↓ Plasma FFA
reset glucose-fatty acid
(Randle) cycle

Liver ↓ Gluconeogenesis

↓ Hyperglycaemia

FFA = free fatty acids

Fig 7.5

Effects of thiazolidinediones on cardiovascular risk factors and markers associated with the metabolic syndrome

TZDs appear to alter many of these factors, possibly via the expression of PPARγ in vascular and other tissues (Fig 7.6). Extensive trials are in progress to determine whether these effects will reduce cardiovascular events in type 2 patients.

Effects of thiazolidinediones on cardiovascular risk factors/markers		
Insulin resistance	Improve insulin sensitivity in type 2 diabetes.	
Hyperinsulinaemia	Reduce fasting hyperinsulinaemia and decrease proportion of proinsulin.	
Abdominal obesity	Visceral depots generally little changed: increase in subcutaneous adipose depots.	
Hyperglycaemia	Improve glycaemic control in type 2 diabetes.	
	Reduce incidence of type 2 diabetes in women with previous gestational diabetes.	
Dyslipidaemia	Pioglitazone and rosiglitazone:	↓FFA
		↑HDL-C
		↑Proportion of larger more buoyant LDL particles
	Pioglitazone:	↓Serum triglycerides
		↓LDL-C
Hypertension	Possible small ↓systolic and diastolic BP.	
Pro-coagulant state	Some antithrombotic effects, (e.g. ↓PAI-1, ↓fibrinogen).	
Inflammation	Decrease some markers, e.g. ↓C-reactive protein.	
Atherosclerosis	Decrease some markers of atherosclerosis (e.g. ↓metalloproteinases, ↓homocysteine, ↓vascular smooth muscle proliferation).	
Albuminuria	Decrease microalbuminuria.	

FFA – *free fatty acid*
HDL-C – *high density lipoprotein cholesterol*
LDL-C – *low density lipoprotein cholesterol*
PAI-1 – *plasminogen activator-1*

Fig 7.6

Thiazolidinediones: indications

Type 2 diabetes
non-obese or obese

First-line monotherapy
*when there is inadequate
glycaemic control by
non-pharmacological measures
+
intolerance/contraindication
to metformin (particularly in
overweight i.e. BMI >25).*

Second-line drug therapy
*when monotherapy with other
agents plus non-pharmacological
measures do not achieve
adequate glycaemic control.*

In combination with:
– Metformin
  *especially in overweight and
  obesity.*

– Sulphonylurea or meglitinide
  *if a metformin/sulphonylurea
  combination is unsuitable.*

Fig 7.7

Additional points

1. Current licencing issues

Current labelling implies that a TZD may be helpful as a last chance use of oral combination therapy before initiating insulin. Individuals with uncontrolled and rising hyperglycaemia who do not respond adequately to a metformin/sulphonylurea combination are unlikely to respond better if one of these agents is substituted with a TZD. Moreover, the slow onset of action of a TZD may result in further loss of control. Use of a TZD is more likely to be effective in early combination therapy.

2. Combination with insulin

In Europe, thiazolidinediones are not indicated for use with insulin, probably due to possible exacerbation of fluid retention, although studies in other countries have shown that thiazolidinediones can substantially reduce insulin requirements.

Thiazolidinediones: precautions, interactions, contraindications

Precautions

– Observe contraindications.

– Monitor:

Liver function before treatment, at intervals during the first year of treatment (e.g. 2-monthly in Europe), and periodically thereafter. Avoid TZD use with liver disease +/or ALT level >2.5 x ULN. If ALT rises >3 times ULN during treatment, observe and stop TZD if ALT level does not quickly fall.

Haemoglobin and stop TZD if severe anaemia supervenes.

Oedema and treat or withdraw TZD as appropriate.

– Special vigilance in elderly/young
(studies in the young have not been conducted).

Ovulation can restart in anovulatory polycystic ovary syndrome (PCOS).
Contraceptive awareness in pre-menopausal PCOS patients.

Drug interactions

Both TZDs are highly protein-bound but no significant interactions with other protein-bound drugs have been reported.

Rosiglitazone
metabolism mainly by CYP2C8 (not a widely used P450 isoform)

Unusual (interactions with paclitaxel, gemfibrozil and rifampicin).

Pioglitazone
CYP3A4 metabolism has the potential to interact

Oral contraceptives (ethinyl oestradiol and norethindrone)
Prescribers should ensure appropriate contraception is explained.
Nifedipine
Many other drugs metabolised by CYP3A4
– no clinically significant interactions reported

Contraindications

Congestive cardiac failure or history of CCF
(New York Heart Association stages I to IV).
Hepatic impairment (e.g. serum ALT >2.5 x ULN) or known liver disease.
Known hypersensitivity to drug.
Pregnancy and breast-feeding.

Not licensed with insulin (some countries).

ALT – *alanine transaminase*
ULN – *upper limit of normal*
PCOS – *polycystic ovary syndrome*
CCF – *congestive cardiac failure*

Fig 7.8

Additional points

1. The main exclusion is evidence of or a history of cardiac failure. This reflects TZD-associated fluid retention with measurable oedema in 5 - 10% of patients. The oedema may respond to a thiazide diuretic, or in those who are not successfully treated it is appropriate to withdraw the drug. This effect appears to be similar for both TZDs in current use, so there is no advantage in switching between them. The oedema is usually accompanied by a dilutional anaemia, and haemoglobin levels may decline by up to 1 mg/dL over 3 - 6 months but level out thereafter.

2. Exclusion due to hepatic impairment is a precaution due to hepatotoxicity experienced with the previously withdrawn troglitazone.

Thiazolidinediones: starting therapy

Monotherapy

- Monotherapy is indicated in overweight or obese individuals (BMI >25) unable to achieve adequate glycaemic control with non-pharmacological measures who are intolerant or have a contraindication to metformin.

Titration steps

1. Introduce thiazolidinedione at lower daily dose (4 mg rosiglitazone; 15 mg or 30 mg pioglitazone).
   Monitor glycaemic control by fasting plasma glucose at clinic visits and patient self-monitoring.

2. Increase dose after 4 - 8 weeks if required to achieve desired level of glycaemic control.

3. If the titration step does not improve control or achieve desired control after 3 months consider an alternative treatment (either substitution or combination therapy).

4. Check liver function at intervals during the first year (e.g. 2-monthly in Europe) and periodically thereafter.

5. If significant uncontrolled oedema occurs or serum ALT >3 x ULN, discontinue the TZD and consider another treatment.

Combination therapy

- Considered when monotherapy with another oral agent does not achieve or maintain adequate glycaemic control.

- Current licencing in Europe also recommends that a metformin/sulphonylurea combination be considered in preference to use of a TZD. It is suggested that a TZD should be used only if there is a contraindication or other reason (e.g. intolerance or hypoglycaemia) why metformin or a sulphonylurea is inappropriate.

- Clinical experience suggests that early use of a TZD in combination therapy is likely to be more effective than delaying until glycaemic control has seriously deteriorated.

Titration steps: adding a thiazolidinedione

If monotherapy with metformin or a sulphonylurea, **and** *use of a metformin/sulphonylurea combination is not appropriate:*

1. Maintain the monotherapy at the minimum dose that produces maximum effect.

2. Introduce thiazolidinedione at lower daily dose (4 mg rosiglitazone; 15 mg or 30 mg pioglitazone).

   Monitor glycaemic control by fasting plasma glucose at clinic visits and patient self-monitoring.

3. Increase dose after 4 - 8 weeks to achieve desired level of glycaemic control (rosiglitazone only licensed for lower dose of 4 mg daily with a sulphonylurea).

4. If the titration step does not improve control or achieve desired control after 3 months consider an alternative treatment.

5. Check liver function at intervals during the first year (e.g. 2-monthly in Europe) and periodically thereafter.

6. If significant uncontrolled oedema occurs or serum ALT rises to >3 x ULN, discontinue the TZD and consider another treatment.

Titration steps: switching to a thiazolidinedione

If a metformin/sulphonylurea combination is achieving glycaemic control but becomes inappropriate (e.g. patient develops a contraindication or intolerance or hypoglycaemia):

1. Stop the offending component of the existing combination.

2. Replace with the lower daily dose of TZD.

3. Increase the dose of TZD after 4 - 8 weeks to achieve desired level of glycaemic control.

If metformin is to be replaced due to intolerance, the above procedure may leave the patient uncontrolled for months and there is a risk that the TZD may not then regain adequate control:

1. Consider off-label triple therapy during the switch period.

2. Explain to patient the purpose of this manoeuvre and explain that the licence states that there is no experience of use of the TZD in triple combination with other oral agents.

3. If patient gives informed consent, record this in notes.

4. Halve the dose of metformin (intolerance may remit) and introduce an equivalent dose of TZD (e.g. if metformin dose is being halved from 2,000 to 1,000 mg daily, introduce 4 mg rosiglitazone or 15 mg pioglitazone).

5. Monitor fasting plasma glucose and titrate up TZD if glycaemic control deteriorates.

If a sulphonylurea is to be replaced for any reason (contraindication or hypoglycaemia) or metformin is to be replaced due to a contraindication:

1. It may not be appropriate to slowly titrate down the existing agent while slowly titrating up the TZD.

2. In this situation, it may be appropriate to switch to the estimated equivalent dose of TZD (which may be the maximum dose) and monitor glucose control carefully.

Check liver function in all uses of a TZD.

Loss of glycaemic control

If glycaemic control is not achieved or sustained with maximally effective doses of a metformin/sulphonylurea combination, it is very unlikely that switching one of these agents for a TZD will obviate the need for insulin.

Thiazolidinediones: efficacy

The blood glucose-lowering effect of a thiazolidinedione is more gradual than other agents and may take 1 - 3 months to achieve full effect.

Monotherapy:

HbA1c	↓ 0.6 - 2.0%
Fasting plasma glucose	↓ 2 - 3 mmol/L

Thiazolidinedione combination (+ metformin or sulphonylurea):

Produces an additive blood glucose-lowering effect:

HbA1c	↓ 1 - 3%
Fasting plasma glucose	↓ 2 - 5 mmol/L

- Due to the gradual glucose-lowering effect of thiazolidinediones, the titration steps are slower than with other oral antidiabetic agents.

- Slightly reduce basal insulin concentrations.

- Hypoglycaemia:

  – Unlikely with TZD/metformin combination.

  – May occur with TZD/sulphonylurea combination.

  The UKPDS established that the progression of type 2 diabetes was delayed for several years by treatment with metformin or a sulphonylurea. Studies are presently in progress to assess the long-term durability of the antihyperglycaemic efficacy of TZDs. Pre-clinical evidence of effects of TZDs on beta-cells has prompted long-term clinical studies that are presently ongoing.

Lipid effects

- Both rosiglitazone and pioglitazone:

  – ↓ Free fatty acid concentrations.

  – ↑ HDL-C by 5 - 15%.

- Pioglitazone produces a reduction in serum triglyceride concentrations (typically 10 - 25%) and has little effect on total cholesterol or LDL-C (low density lipoprotein cholesterol).

- Rosiglitazone appears to be less likely to reduce total triglyceride concentrations and usually produces a small increase in total cholesterol and LDL-C which stabilises after 3 - 6 months (typical increase up to about 0.5 mmol/L). Both TZDs appear to increase the proportion of larger more buoyant (less atherogenic) LDL particles, and reduce the proportion of the smaller denser LDL.

- Drugs with inherent hyperglycaemic effects (e.g. glucocorticoids) may require an increase in TZD dosage.

Thiazolidinediones: adverse effects

Fluid retention	General feature of thiazolidinedione PPARγ agonists, hence caution in cardiac failure.
	Probably dose-dependent.
	Oedema (5 - 10% of patients).
	Some oedema patients respond to a thiazide diuretic.
	Despite the fluid retention, little change has been noted in blood pressure other than a very small reduction in both systolic and diastolic. No significant adverse cardiac events have been reported (e.g. no cardiac hypertrophy).
Dilutional anaemia	Associated with fluid retention.
	Decrease in haemoglobin of up to 1 g/dL not unusual – levels out 3 - 6 months.
Hepatic impairment	Fatal cases of idiosyncratic hepatotoxicity with previous TZD troglitazone (withdrawn from use).
	Fatal hepatotoxicity not been found with rosiglitazone or pioglitazone (isolated cases of abnormal liver function).
	Regular monitoring of liver function (e.g. serum ALT) advised.
Weight gain	2 - 4 kg. Not uncommon during first 6 months of treatment. Weight appears to stabilise thereafter.
	Due to: – Mostly attributed to extra adipose tissue (peripheral subcutaneous) and not in visceral depots; appears to reflect the adipogenic effect of PPARγ activation. *– Extra fluid.*
Hypoglycaemia	Clinically significant only with combination (TZD plus an insulin-releaser).

Fig 7.9

Thiazolidinediones at a glance

Class	Thiazolidinediones
Action	Improve insulin action

Indications	• *Type 2 diabetes*
	  – Monotherapy if metformin not appropriate
	  – Combination with metformin or a
	    sulphonylurea (or meglitinide)[a]

Choice	If either metformin or a sulphonylurea is not appropriate for combination therapy
Treatment	Start with lower dose and titrate very slowly over 4 - 8 weeks to the higher dose if required[b] – Rosiglitazone start 4 mg/day; max 8 mg/day – Pioglitazone start 15 mg/day or 30 mg/day; max 45 mg/day
Cautions and contraindications	Cardiac failure or history of cardiac failure Impaired liver function Pregnancy and breast-feeding Combination with insulin
Efficacy	HbA1c $\downarrow$ 0.6 - 2.0% FPG $\downarrow$ 2 - 3 mmol/L – Not cause serious hypoglycaemia with metformin – Can improve lipid profile – Reduced thrombotic factors – Reduced basal hyperinsulinaemia – Reduced albuminuria
Adverse effects	Fluid retention leading to oedema and dilutional anaemia Weight gain Hypoglycaemia when combined with a sulphonylurea
Precautions	Check for cardiac contraindications Monitor liver function (e.g. serum ALT) Rosiglitazone interacts with paclitaxel, gemfibrozil and rifampicin; pioglitazone has possible interactions with oral contraception and drugs metabolised by CYP3A4 Possible restart of ovulation in PCOS

[a] Assumes inadequate glycaemic control with metformin or a sulphonylurea
as monotherapy.
[b] Up to 4 mg daily rosiglitazone with a sulphonylurea.

Rosiglitazone-metformin single-tablet combination

A single-tablet combination of rosiglitazone and metformin is available in two strengths (rosiglitazone-metformin: 1 mg/500 mg and rosiglitazone-metformin: 2 mg/500 mg).

Rosiglitazone-metformin: pharmacokinetics

- Pharmacokinetics of each agent is unaltered by the presence of the other (see Figs 6.2 and 7.2).

Rosiglitazone-metformin: mode of action

- Both rosiglitazone and metformin are *antihyperglycaemic* agents which increase the action of insulin.

- The cellular mechanisms of action of rosiglitazone and metformin are different and complementary, enabling them to be used in combination with approximately additive glucose-lowering efficacy.

- The glucose-lowering efficacy of both rosiglitazone and metformin requires the presence of insulin but neither agent raises basal insulin concentrations.

- Both rosiglitazone and metformin exert various effects on cardiovascular risk factors and markers associated with the metabolic syndrome (see Figs 6.6 and 7.6).

Rosiglitazone-metformin combination: indications

Type 2 diabetes	Second-line drug therapy
non-obese or obese	*when monotherapy with metformin is inadequate in achieving glycaemic control especially in overweight and obesity.*
	When current therapy comprises a combination of rosiglitazone and metformin as separate tablets if the single-tablet combination is more convenient.
	Possible transfer of combination of metformin and a sulphonylurea if the sulphonylurea component is no longer tolerated, becomes contraindicated, or patient suffers uncontrollable episodes of hypoglycaemia.

Fig 7.10

Rosiglitazone-metformin: starting therapy

1. If patient is inadequately controlled on metformin alone:
   - Maintain existing dosage of metformin and add 1 mg rosiglitazone per 500 mg metformin.
   - Increase to 2 mg rosiglitazone per 500 mg of metformin after 4 - 8 weeks if required to achieve glycaemic control.
2. If switching from rosiglitazone and metformin as separate tablets:
   - Select the nearest rosiglitazone-metformin dosage match.
3. Transferring from a metformin-sulphonylurea combination:
   - Suggest gradually decrease sulphonylurea while titrating up rosiglitazone-metformin:
     – Starting at 1 mg rosiglitazone per 500 mg metformin.

Additional point

1. Rosiglitazone-metformin is unlikely to give better glycaemic control in conditions of so-called 'sulphonylurea failure' when beta-cell function is already very severely depleted.

Rosiglitazone-metformin: efficacy

The efficacy of rosiglitazone-metformin is the same as rosiglitazone plus metformin as separate tablets, i.e. approximately additive glucose-lowering effect but slowly generated (provided that there is sufficient beta-cell function to maintain insulin secretion).

HbA1c	↓ 1 - 3%
Fasting plasma glucose	↓ 2 - 5 mmol/L

- Likely to slightly reduce basal insulin concentrations and some lipid parameters (FFA and VLDL-TG)
- May increase HDL and large buoyant LDL-C

Rosiglitazone-metformin: precautions (see Figs 6.8 and 7.8)

- Same as *both* rosiglitazone and metformin.
- Note especially the exclusion of patients with cardiac failure and impaired renal function.
- Appreciate risk of oedema and rare risk of lactic acidosis.
- Remember need to monitor liver function and serum creatinine.

Rosiglitazone-metformin: adverse effects (see Figs 6.9 and 7.9)

- Slight weight gain.
- Unlikely to cause significant hypoglycaemia.

Rosiglitazone-metformin in combination at a glance*

Combination	Rosiglitazone (thiazolidinedione) and metformin (biguanide)
Action	Improve insulin action by complementary mechanisms
Indications	● *Type 2 diabetes* Second-line drug therapy if metformin alone or a metformin/sulphonylurea combination is not appropriate
Dosage strengths	1 mg/500 mg and 2 mg/500 mg (rosiglitazone/metformin)
Treatment	Start 1 mg/500 mg once-daily titrated up to maximum four-times daily: then 2 mg/500 mg titrated up to four-times daily
Main cautions and contraindications	Cardiac failure, history of cardiac failure Renal impairment, liver disease Combination with insulin
Efficacy	HbA1c ↓1 - 3% FPG ↓2 - 5 mmol/L
Adverse effects	No serious hypoglycaemia Risk of oedema, dilutional anaemia and gastrointestinal symptoms Rare risk of lactic acidosis
Precautions	Check liver and renal function Can restart ovulation in PCOS Possible interactions with cimetidine, paclitaxel, gemfibrozil and rifampicin

* See separate summaries for rosiglitazone (page 81) and metformin (page 66) – cautions, contraindications, precautions and adverse effects for *both* apply.

Historical background

1909	Jean de Meyer names "insuline" from pancreas.
1921	Banting (physician and surgeon) and Best (student) in Toronto discover that insulin ("extracts of pancreas") lowers glucose in pancreatectomised dog.
1922	Leonard Thompson (aged 14 yrs) – first patient to be treated with insulin.
1920s	Short-acting bovine and porcine pancreas extracts.
1930s	Improved purification of insulin.
1936	Hagedorn shows prolonged effects of insulin bound with protamine, a protein from fish sperm.
1946	Isophane (NPH- Neutral Protamine Hagedorn) insulin introduced into clinical practice.
1955	Sanger identifies amino acid sequence of insulin.
1970s	Highly purified (monocomponent) insulins.
1980s	Biosynthetic human insulin.
	Premixed biphasic insulins.
	Insulin pumps for CSII (continuous subcutaneous insulin infusion).
	Pen injection devices.
1990s	Rapid-acting insulin analogues.
2000s	Long-acting insulin analogues.

- Insulin is a polypeptide hormone with 51 amino acids arranged in two chains (*A-chain*, 21 amino acids: *B-chain*, 30 amino acids), linked by two disulphide bridges between cysteine residues.

- The amino acid sequence of the B-chain strongly influences binding to the insulin receptor (especially amino acid residues B12, B16 and B23 - 25). Receptor binding leads to the biological effects of insulin.

- Insulin has anabolic effects on glucose, lipid and protein metabolism and facilitates growth and cellular differentiation.

- Insulin replacement therapy is used when there is no endogenous insulin or significant insulin deficiency.

- Insulin preparations differ in source:

  – *Bovine* or *porcine* pancreas extracts.

  – Human *biosynthetic* produced by recombinant DNA in yeast (pyr) or E.coli bacteria (prb and crb).

  – *Semisynthetic* – porcine insulin altered chemically into the human insulin sequence (emp).

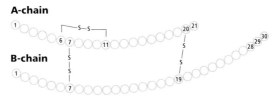

A-chain

B-chain

[Key amino acids: A8-Thr, A10-Ile, A21-Asn, B28-Pro, B29-Lys, B30-Thr]

Fig 8.1 Structure of human insulin

Amino acid substitutions in natural and analogue insulins	
Insulin source/type	**Amino acid alterations**
Natural	
Synthetic human insulin	Same as endogenous human insulin (Fig 8.1)
Porcine insulin	B30-Ala
Beef insulin	A8-Ala
	A10-Val
	B30-Ala
Analogue	
Insulin Aspart	B28-Asp
Insulin Lispro	B28-Lys
	B29-Pro
Insulin Glargine	A21-Gly
	B31-Arg
	B32-Arg
Insulin Detemir	B29-Lys is acylated with a C14 fatty acid side chain (myristic acid)
	B30-threonine deletion

Fig 8.2

- Insulin preparations differ in the time of onset and duration of action, depending on their amino acid sequence, and formulation with protamine and/or zinc.

- All insulins are rapidly degraded in the circulation and after receptor binding and internalisation by target cells, especially liver: some insulin is eliminated via bile and urine.

- *Insulin analogues* are biosynthetic insulins in which the amino acid sequence has been modified to alter the pharmacokinetic properties, which affect onset and duration of action.
- All insulins are highly purified and are available in concentrations of 100 units per ml or *U-100* (1 unit of activity is equivalent to 38.5 μg [6 nmol] of purified human insulin).

Insulin: pharmacokinetics

	(i) Basal insulins	
	Natural insulin suspensions	**Basal insulin analogues**
Bioavailability/ absorption	Non-covalent complexes of insulin with *protamine* or *zinc* delay absorption and prolong action:	Basal insulin analogues do not use either zinc or protamine for their prolonged action.
	Isophane insulins Addition of protamine (neutral protamine Hagedorn – NPH)	*Insulin Glargine†* Formulated in acid solution (pH 4.0). Following injection into subcutaneous tissue (neutral pH), microprecipitates occur which slow absorption and delay clearance, resulting in prolongation of action.
	Lente insulins* Insulin-zinc suspensions	Released at a steady rate from subcutaneous injection site – after about 90 minutes a peakless plateau is achieved (lasts for over 24 hours).
		Insulin Detemir† Self-association prolongs subcutaneous absorption with further prolongation due to reversible binding (via its fatty acid chain) to albumin in plasma.
	* These formulations have wide variations in time to peak insulin concentration and the peak concentration achieved.	*† Analogue insulins require no resuspension which also reduces the variability in absorption. This better reflects the physiological insulin profile and is associated with reduced hypoglycaemia (particularly nocturnal).*

Fig 8.3

(ii) Bolus insulins

	Natural insulins	**Rapid-acting insulin analogues**

Bioavailability/ absorption

Subcutaneous injection

Natural insulins in solution associate into hexamers which retards absorption.

Before absorption into the circulation, the hexamers dissociate into dimers and then monomers – results in a delay before plasma insulin concentration reaches a peak (often after 2 hours for short-acting insulins) which does not coincide with the peak post-meal glucose (which usually occurs at 1 hour).

Time course of action of biosynthetic 'human' insulin is more predictable than animal-derived insulins, in part due to the reduced frequency of aller-gy and antibody formation.

All animal-derived insulins are highly purified with reduced proinsulin (the main contami-nant after extraction from the pancreas) which has improved the pharmacological specificity.

Intravenous infusion

Good bioavailability with i.v. infusion.
Half-life 2 - 5 minutes.

Subcutaneous injection

When injected subcutaneously, these analogues are monomeric and therefore more rapidly absorbed, avoiding absorption problems from dimerisation and hexamerisation of short-acting (regular, neutral) human insulin.

Fig 8.4

Classification of insulins

Pragmatic classification of subcutaneous insulins

Insulin category	Alternative 'name'	Duration of action
Basal	'Background'	Intermediate-acting
	'Maintenance'	Long-acting
Bolus	'Prandial'	Rapid-acting
	'Meal'	Short-acting
Biphasic	'Pre-mixed'	Pre-mixed combination of
	'Mixtures'	Rapid-acting + isophane (NPH)
		or
		Short-acting + isophane (NPH)

Fig 8.5

Duration of action of subcutaneous insulins

	Time of onset	Peak	Duration of action
Basal insulins			
Intermediate or long-acting	1 - 8 h	2 - 20 h	10 - 24+ h
Bolus insulins			
Rapid-acting	10 min	1 - 3 h	3 - 4 h
Short-acting	30 - 60 min	1 - 5 h	6 - 8 h
Biphasic insulins			
Pre-mixed	10 - 30 min	1 - 12 h	10 - 24 h

Fig 8.6

Basal insulins

- Time course of lente insulins is slightly slower than isophane insulins. Ultralente has a longer duration of action due to the high zinc levels and crystal size.

- The insulin analogues have a long duration of action due to their physiochemical properties.

Bolus insulins

- Short-acting insulins – *regular (neutral)* human insulins – are natural insulins with a fast onset and short duration of action.

- Rapid-acting insulin *analogues* have a faster onset of action and shorter duration of action compared to regular short-acting human insulins. Rapid-acting insulins have a similar kinetic profile to endogenous insulin concentrations after a meal.

Insulin: subcutaneous regimens

Basal-bolus regimens

- A basal-bolus regimen offers a close approximation to an endogenous insulin profile. Administration of a pre-bedtime long-acting insulin covers overnight insulin requirements as well as daytime background, with supplementation of pre-meal bolus insulins (either rapid- or short-acting insulin).

Biphasic insulins

- Biphasic insulins consist of a pre-mixed combination of a basal insulin (either intermediate- or long-acting insulin) with bolus insulin (either a rapid- or short-acting insulin).

- Administration is usually twice-daily – pre-breakfast and pre-evening meal. The longer-acting insulin gives the basal (background) profile and covers the mid-day meal, while breakfast and evening meals are covered by the bolus insulins.

- Initial peak action is determined by the quantity of bolus insulin in the mixture. Altering the proportion of bolus insulin in the preparation may not always improve glycaemic control due to hypoglycaemic episodes.

Additional points

1. *Soluble (clear)* is still used to describe *regular (neutral)* insulin. This nomenclature is now outmoded since long-acting insulin analogues are also soluble (clear).

2. *Cloudy* insulins contain intermediate- or long-acting formulations.

3. The visual distinction of clear and cloudy insulins can still be helpful to patients who prepare their own mixture of isophane with a short- or rapid-acting insulin (see page 102).

Time course profiles of insulin effects
Subcutaneous injection

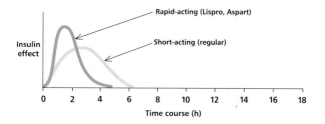

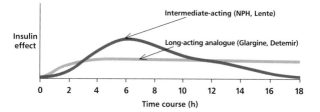

Biphasic mixture

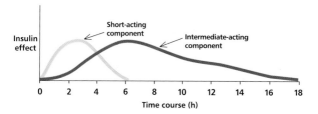

Fig 8.7

Basal-bolus regimens
Subcutaneous injection

Arrows show times of insulin injections

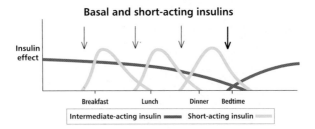

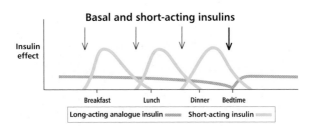

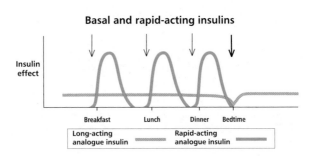

Fig 8.8

Insulin: mode of action

Insulin therapy aims to mimic the physiological profile of endogenous insulin. Tailoring therapy to the individual involves selection of appropriate insulin formulation and administration regimen.

Main metabolic effects of insulin	
Glucose effects	Suppression of hepatic glucose output.
	Stimulation of peripheral glucose utilisation.
	Glucose uptake into muscle and fat
Lipid effects	Increase lipid uptake and storage.
	Decrease lipid mobilisation.
Protein effects	Increase amino acid uptake and protein synthesis.

Fig 8.9

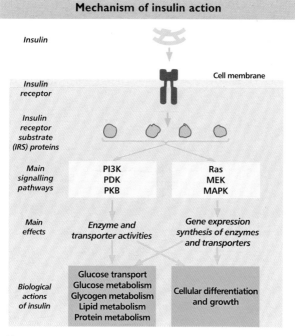

Mechanism of insulin action

PI3K – phosphatidylinositol 3-kinase
PDK – phosphoinositide dependent kinase
PKB (=akt) – protein kinase B

Ras – rat sarcoma protein
MAPK – mitogen-activated protein kinase
MEK – mitogen-activated protein kinase kinase

Fig 8.10

Insulin preparations

Insulins are dispensed as a solution with either phenol or cresol (a transport vehicle) in glass vials or cartridges. Storage should usually be in a refrigerator (2 - 8°C). Temperature and light can affect stability in solution.

Insulin within the vials/bottles is drawn-up using a needle and syringe: cartridges are inserted into pen injector devices or infusion pumps, or already inserted in pre-filled pen injector devices.

The insulin solutions are either *monophasic* preparations – either basal or bolus preparation – or *biphasic* which are pre-mixed combinations.

Biphasic mixtures (pre-mixed combinations)	
Biphasic mixtures	*Usually labelled according to the relative proportion of bolus and basal insulin in the combination.**
European nomenclature	
'30/70'	30% short-acting and 70% intermediate-acting insulin
'50/50'	50% short-acting and 50% intermediate-acting insulin
'10/90'	10% short-acting and 90% intermediate-acting insulin
'25'	25% rapid-acting and 75% intermediate-acting insulin
'30'	30% rapid-acting and 70% intermediate-acting insulin

* In Europe the % of short- or rapid-acting insulin is stated first. By contrast in the USA, the % of long-acting insulin is stated first.

Fig 8.11

Storage of insulin		
	Storage time	
	Refrigerated	*Room temperature*
Vials/bottles		
Unopened vials	Expiry date	1 month
Opened vials	1 - 2 months*	1 month
	* Opened vials lose potency over time, even when refrigerated.	
Cartridges for pens		
Short- or rapid-acting insulins	Expiry date	1 month
Isophane or mixtures	Expiry date	7 days
Disposable pre-filled pens		
Rapid-acting	Expiry date	14 days
Isophane	Expiry date	10 days

Fig 8.12

Modes of insulin delivery

Intravenous infusion of short-acting insulins

- Unmodified short-acting insulins are suitable.
- As the half-life of intravenous insulin resembles that of endogenous insulin (2 - 5 minutes) a constant infusion is required to maintain adequate levels.
- Used in acute illness.
- Requires strict glucose monitoring.

Subcutaneous injection with syringe

- Disposable *plastic syringes* with either 50 unit or 100 unit markings are now in common use. These may have repeated use. Disposable ultrafine (≥ 29 g) needles – between 8 - 12 mm in length – are attached separately.
- *Glass syringes* are uncommonly used. Disadvantages include the need to clean syringe and needle under sterile conditions and breakage risk.

Subcutaneous injection with pen injector device

- Pen injector devices enable the dose to be dialled, use either replaceable cartridges of insulin or are classified as 'disposable' as the insulin cartridge is fixed inside the casing of the device (i.e. 'pre-loaded'). A mechanised dose selection aids administration of accurate volumes.
- Cartridges contain either 1.5 ml or 3.0 ml of U-100 insulin.
- Disposable needles used with these devices are ultrafine (≥ 29 g), 8 - 12 mm in length.

Continuous subcutaneous insulin infusion (CSII) – 'the Insulin Pump'

- The apparatus is a miniature programmable syringe pump with infusion tube connected to a catheter inserted into the subcutaneous tissue (often in the abdomen).
- The programmable pump continuously delivers either short- or rapid-acting insulin via the indwelling subcutaneous catheter. A constant basal infusion rate provides the background insulin requirement. The patient activates additional infusion of boluses to cover the meals.

Procedures for subcutaneous insulin injection

Syringe
1. Shake insulin vial gently and invert.
2. Draw air (equivalent to injection volume) into syringe.
3. Pierce vial cap with needle.
4. Expel air into vial and draw insulin into syringe up to the required dose.
5. Insert needle at 90° to skin surface and inject syringe contents.

Pen injector device
1. Shake pen injector device gently.
2. Errors arising from air bubbles in the needle may be eliminated if 2 - 4 units of insulin are expelled before use.
3. Dial up dose required.
4. Insert needle at 90° to skin surface, inject contents by depressing plunger.

Fig 8.13

Timing of subcutaneous insulin injection

Insulin type	Timing of subcutaneous injections in relation to food intake
Short-acting insulins	Inject 30 - 45 minutes before meals in order to match peak insulin action to prandial glucose absorption. (A delayed meal has the risk of hypoglycaemia).
Rapid-acting insulins	Inject immediately before, during or just after meal.
Intermediate and long-acting insulins	Pre-bedtime long-acting insulin covers overnight insulin requirements as well as daytime background.

Fig 8.14

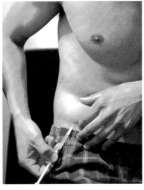

Getty Images/Keith Brofsky

Fig 8.15

Injection sites

- Rotation of injection sites (Fig 8.16) is important to avoid lipo-hypertrophy or lipoatrophy.

- To reduce variation in insulin absorption rates it is often advisable to use similar injection sites for pre-breakfast (e.g. legs) and pre-lunch (e.g. abdomen) rather than a completely random alteration of sites.

- Rates of absorption are more rapid from abdomen than arm, buttock and thigh, and increase with exercise and heat.

- Lipohypertrophy pre-disposes to a non-uniform absorption profile.

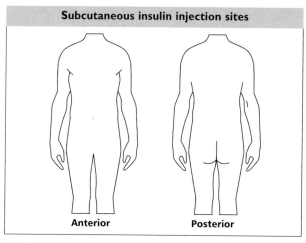

Subcutaneous insulin injection sites

Anterior　　　**Posterior**

Fig 8.16

Factors affecting subcutaneous insulin absorption

- Type of insulin.
- Site of administration.
- Concurrent smoking.
- Exercise.
- Temperature.
- If the injection site is massaged.
- If injection too deep (into muscle), insulin absorption could be more rapid.

Insulin: indications

Insulin: indications	
Type 1 diabetes	At diagnosis.
Type 2 diabetes	Occasionally at presentation with marked hyperglycaemia.
	Poor glycaemic control (e.g. HbA1c >7%) on oral therapies.
	Hyperglycaemic (osmotic) symptoms.
	Marked unintentional weight loss.
	Special circumstances:
	Acute illness (e.g. myocardial infarction or diabetic ketoacidosis).
	Surgery.
	Severe renal or liver disease.
	Painful peripheral neuropathy or amyotrophy.
	Pregnancy (either gestational diabetes or pre-existing diabetes).
	Allergy or intolerance to oral therapies.

Fig 8.17

Selecting an insulin regimen

● **Intensive insulin therapy** can be achieved by either *multiple daily injections of insulin (MDI)* e.g. as basal-bolus and twice-daily biphasic or by *continuous subcutaneous insulin infusion (CSII)*. These regimens are advised for most diabetes patients.

● **Less intense regimens** may be used in the elderly or those in whom the risk of hypoglycaemia may be a major clinical hazard (includes elderly or individuals with multiple co-morbidities, severe arthritis or visual impairment).

● Other factors include social circumstances, life-style, weight and osmotic symptoms.

● *Children* and *adolescents*: intensive insulin regimens are encouraged where practicable and accepted by patient and family.

● Before and during *pregnancy*: patients are advised to follow an intensive insulin regimen where possible.

Subcutaneous insulin regimens

Type of regimen	Patient types	Advantages	Disadvantages
Once-daily			
Long- or intermediate-acting insulin	Often used in elderly type 2 diabetes patients who require insulin to be given by others.	*Simplicity*	*Lack of flexibility* *Often poor control* *Hypoglycaemic episodes*
	First time use of insulin.		
	Short-term intercurrent illness (type 2 diabetes).		
Twice-daily			
Pre-mixed combination intermediate- or long-acting insulin	Type 1 diabetes Type 2 diabetes	*Simplicity*	*Lack of flexibility* *Hypoglycaemic episodes*
Bolus/ pre-prandial only			
Short- or rapid-acting insulin	Type 2 diabetes	*Flexible*	*Multiple injections* *Poor control of fasting glucose*
Basal-bolus			
Pre-bedtime long- or intermediate-acting insulin + pre-meal short- or rapid-acting insulin	Type 1 diabetes Type 2 diabetes	*Flexible*	*Multiple injections* *Hypoglycaemic episodes between meals/night*
Oral therapy +insulin combination	Type 2 diabetes	*Adaptability*	*Multiple administrations* *Precautions with oral agent(s)*
Continuous subcutaneous insulin infusion (CSII)	Type 1 diabetes Type 2 diabetes (see below)	*Reduced insulin dose* *Reduced hypoglycaemia* *Enhanced freedom variability of meals*	*Should not be used without home glucose monitoring or correct motivation* *Catheter site infection*

Fig 8.18

Once-daily insulin therapy

Basal (long- or intermediate-acting) insulin in type 2 diabetes – often administered at bedtime – to suppress overnight glucose production which reduces fasting glycaemia. Combination with oral blood glucose-lowering drug may assist in maintaining glycaemic control.

Pre-prandial insulin only

Occasionally used in acute illness in type 2 diabetes. Does not give good control.

Twice-daily regimens

- Either twice-daily basal insulin or biphasic insulin.
- Requires regularity of life-style and three meals per day, and often snacks between meals to reduce risk of hypoglycaemia.
- Initial peak action is determined by the quantity of bolus insulin in the mixture. Altering the proportion of bolus insulin may not always improve glycaemic control due to hypoglycaemic episodes.

Basal-bolus regimens

- Pre-bedtime long-acting insulin covers overnight and daytime insulin requirements as well as daytime background.
- Pre-meal bolus insulins (either rapid- or short-acting) offer flexibility with regards timing of meals.
- A preferred regimen for intensive insulin therapy.

Continuous subcutaneous insulin infusion (CSII)

- Can be designed to closely mimic endogenous insulin profiles.
- Programmable constant infusion of short- or rapid-acting insulin provides background insulin.
- Patient selects additional infusion of boluses to cover the meals.

Indications for CSII	Uncontrollable glycaemia with conventional regimens.
	Impaired awareness of hypoglycaemia.
	Severe early morning insulin resistance (dawn phenomenon).
	Pregnancy.
	Extreme insulin sensitivity.
	Unpredictable mealtimes.

Fig 8.19

Insulin + oral glucose-lowering therapy in type 2 diabetes

- *Combination of insulin with metformin* in patients already treated with insulin may improve glycaemic control and reduce the weight gain.
- *Combination of insulin with a sulphonylurea* may reduce insulin dose or improve control while beta-cell function lasts. As beta-cell function declines, sulphonylurea effect may be lost and full insulin therapy required.
- *Combination of insulin with a thiazolidinedione* may reduce insulin dose, but this combination is not licensed in Europe. Pioglitazone and rosiglitazone can increase weight and fluid retention, and combination with insulin may increase these side-effects.

Starting insulin therapy

Insulin dose

- Needs to be tailored to the individual patient.
- Usual total dose of insulin for an adult is 0.5 - 1.0 unit/kg body weight per day.
  - Requirements increase with insulin resistance e.g. over-weight/obesity.
  - Lower dose is often needed with renal or liver impairment.
- For basal-bolus regimen:
  - Approx ½ of total daily dose as basal (either once-daily or divided between morning and evening).
  - Approx ½ of total daily dose divided between meal-related bolus injections.
- For biphasic regimen:
  - Approx ½ to ⅔ of total daily dose with breakfast.
  - Approx ½ or ⅓ of total daily dose before or with evening meal.

Starting dose for adults

- Start with low dose e.g. 10 - 12 units per day, with gradual up-titration to avoid hypoglycaemia.
- Monitor fasting, preprandial or postprandial glucose.
- Titrate up by 2 - 4 units per day to achieve target control.
- Starting insulin in pregnancy and during acute treatment of myocardial infarction should only be undertaken by specialists.

Starting dose for children

- Should only be undertaken by specialists.
- Requires prior management of acute presentation.
- Usually start at 0.1 units/kg body weight per day: up-titrate very carefully.
- Special education and support for child and family.

Patient education is key to successful insulin treatment

- Explain general principles, advantages, precautions and life-style adjustments associated with insulin therapy.
- Explain selection of insulin injection devices and appropriate size of needles. Some individuals start with pen injector device rather than syringe and needle. Pen injectors are useful with a basal-bolus regimen.

- Familiarise patient with name/type of insulin: demonstrate procedure to draw up/dial up measured dose of insulin.
- Demonstrate correct injection technique with rotation of injection sites.
- Discuss life-style – regularity and composition of meals, snacks and exercise.
- Ensure awareness of hypoglycaemia and its treatment.
- Give advice about adjustment of dose if glucose levels are high e.g. due to illness.
- Provide further information regarding special circumstances such as driving, holidays.

Psychological support when starting insulin

- To allay anxieties about the need for insulin.
- Needle phobia (most needle injections do not hurt).

Mixing insulins		
• Short-acting preparation must be drawn into syringe before longer-acting insulin to avoid contamination of short-acting vial with either zinc or protamine.		
Combining insulin preparations		**Practical considerations**
Rapid-acting analogue	+ isophane	- Mixture stable in any ratio. - Administer immediately after mixing.
Short-acting	+ isophane	- Mixture stable in any ratio. - Pre-filling is acceptable. - Patient-prepared syringes stable for at least 1 month if refrigerated.
Short-acting	+ lente	- Binding of regular insulin begins immediately and continues for 24 h. - Activity of short-acting insulin is blunted. - Interval between mixing the insulins and administering the injection should be standardised but administer immediately after mixing if possible.
Glargine		- Cannot be mixed with other insulins.
Detemir		- Cannot be mixed with other insulins.

Fig 8.20

Additional point

1. Rapid-acting Aspart can be mixed with NPH, but it is advised to use pre-mixed cartridges or pen of NovoMix. Lispro can only be mixed as supplied in pre-mixed cartridges or pen of Humalog Mix.

Insulin: adverse effects

Insulin: adverse effects		
Hypoglycaemia	Type 1 diabetes – more common	
	Type 2 diabetes – less common	Often have relative preservation of hormonal response to hypoglycaemia. May have more 'physiological' insulin profiles due to the presence of endogenous insulin.
	Increased with duration of therapy	*Exacerbating factors:* *- Missed meal* *- Alcohol excess* *- Exercise* *- Malabsorption* *- Eating disorders* *- Insulin pharmacokinetics (change from animal to human insulin)* *- Pharmacodynamic factors (e.g. decline in renal function with reduced insulin metabolism)* *- Changes in insulin sensitivity (e.g. hypopituitism, hypothyroidism, Addison's disease)*
Weight gain	Variable 2 - 4 kg. *Greater in some patients with type 2 diabetes.*	Due to a decrease in urinary glucose loss, anabolic effects of insulin, and changes in appetite. Regimens which combine metformin are associated with less weight gain.
Lipohypertrophy	Localised subcutaneous adipose tissue from frequent use of the same injection site.	Considered to be due to localised high concentrations of insulin producing enhanced adipogenesis. May alter insulin absorption from site. Treatment includes avoidance of the site and use of other injection sites.
Lipoatrophy	Due to localised immune response to impurities of the insulin solution.	Rare with highly purified and biosynthetic insulins.
Allergy	Local allergic reactions Generalised allergic reactions	Uncommon Rare

Fig 8.21

Additional factors when starting insulin therapy include:

- Anxiety.
- Needle phobia.
- Minor injection site bleeding/bruising – often due to poor technique or the use of longer needles.

Nocturnal hypoglycaemia

This may go unrecognised. May be due to the kinetic profile of evening insulins.

Easy measures to correct this include a pre-bed snack, reduced alcohol, reducing the dose of evening insulin. Other treatment choices include use of a rapid-acting insulin analogue instead of regular short-acting insulin, or achieving a flatter basal profile with a long-acting analogue instead of other basal insulins.

Insulin species and hypoglycaemia risk

A few individuals experience reduced intensity or even loss of symptoms of hypoglycaemia when changed from animal-derived to biosynthetic human insulin therapy. Minor differences in pharmacokinetics or the presence of high titres of anti-insulin antibodies have been implicated. Reverting back to the original species of insulin may, in some of these cases, restore the hypoglycaemic symptom awareness.

Self-monitoring of capillary blood glucose

Patient education will include information about recognising and responding to early symptoms of hypoglycaemia. Self-monitoring of capillary blood glucose should be encouraged (see Fig 2.5, page 15), especially to confirm symptoms of low blood glucose.

Patients should inform partners and colleagues

Patients should be encouraged to carry identification that they have diabetes, as well as a supply of glucose. Patients should inform partners and colleagues about the features of hypoglycaemia and the intervention required.

Treatment of insulin-induced hypoglycaemia

Onset of symptoms (mild symptoms):

At least 20 g of oral carbohydrate

e.g.   7 dextrose tablets

4 teaspoons of sugar/3 teaspoons of honey

115 ml (½ bottle) of lucozade

This may be repeated.

Severe symptoms (assistance from another person required):

1. Buccal glucose gel (Hypostop) – variable efficacy

2. i.v. infusion 20% dextrose (100 ml) via a large cannulated vein
   (i.v. infusion 50% dextrose [25 - 50 ml] is widely used, but is best avoided due to the hazard from extravasation, tissue necrosis and thrombophlebitis)

3. Glucagon 1 mg (i.v. infusion, i.m. injection)

   Avoid in type 2 diabetes as beta-cells may secrete more insulin.

   If recovery is fast – follow with a snack to keep blood glucose high.

   After recovery: precipitating factors (e.g. missed meal/alcohol excess) should be identified to avoid recurrence.

Fig 8.22

Delayed recovery from hypoglycaemia

- If the hypoglycaemia is severe or prolonged.

- Alternative cause of altered consciousness e.g. stroke, drug over-dose or alcohol excess.

- Post-ictal state following seizure from neuroglycopenia.

Classification and characteristics of insulins

(i) Basal insulins			
Name	**Manufacturer**	**Structure**	**Vial, cartridge or pen**
Intermediate- and long-acting insulins			
Insulatard	*Novo Nordisk*	Human	Vial, cartridge, pre-loaded pe
Humulin I	*Lilly*	Human	Vial, cartridge, pre-loaded pe
Hypurin Bovine Isophane	*CP Pharmaceuticals*	Beef	Vial and cartridge
Hypurin Bovine Lente	*CP Pharmaceuticals*	Beef	Vial
Hypurin Bovine PZI	*CP Pharmaceuticals*	Beef	Vial
Hypurin Porcine Isophane	*CP Pharmaceuticals*	Pork	Vial and cartridge
Isuman Basal	*Aventis Pharma*	Human	Vial, cartridge, pre-loaded pe
Monotard	*Novo Nordisk*	Human	Vial
Pork Insulatard	*Novo Nordisk*	Pork	Vial
Ultratard	*Novo Nordisk*	Human	Vial
Lantus (glargine)	*Aventis Pharma*	Analogue	Vial, cartridge, pre-loaded pe
Levemir (detemir)	*Novo Nordisk*	Analogue	Vial, cartridge, pre-loaded pe

Fig 8.23

(ii) Bolus insulins			
Name	**Manufacturer**	**Structure**	**Vial, cartridge or pen**
Rapid-acting insulins			
NovoRapid (Aspart)	*Novo Nordisk*	Analogue	Vial, cartridge, pre-loaded p
Humalog (Lispro)	*Lilly*	Analogue	Vial, cartridge, pre-loaded p
Short-acting insulins			
Actrapid	*Novo Nordisk*	Human	Vial, cartridge, pre-loaded p
Velosulin	*Novo Nordisk*	Human	Vial
Humulin S	*Lilly*	Human	Vial, cartridge, pre-loaded p
Hypurin Bovine Neutral	*CP Pharmaceuticals*	Beef	Vial and cartridge
Hypurin Porcine Neutral	*CP Pharmaceuticals*	Pork	Vial and cartridge
Insuman Rapid	*Aventis Pharma*	Human	Cartridge, pre-loaded pen
Pork Actrapid	*Novo Nordisk*	Pork	Vial

Fig 8.24

Timing of administration	Onset (h)	Peak (h)	Duration of action (h)
~30 min before a meal or bedtime	1	2 - 12	16 - 22
"	1	2 - 8	10 - 16
"	1 - 4	6 - 12	16 - 22
"	2 - 6	8 - 12	18 - 24+
"	4 - 8	8 - 20	24+
"	1 - 4	6 - 12	16 - 22
"	1	2 - 4	12 - 18
"	1 - 2	3 - 12	18 - 24
"	1 - 2	2 - 1	18 - 24
"	2 - 4	8 - 20	24+
Anytime once-daily (occasionally twice-daily)	2 - 4	4 - 20	24+
~30 min before a meal or bedtime	2 - 4	6 - 8	18 - 24

Timing of administration	Onset	Peak (h)	Duration of action (h)
- 15 min before or during a meal	10 min	1 - 3	3 - 4
"	10 min	1 - 2	3 - 4
5 - 30 min before a meal	30 min	2 - 3	6 - 8
"	30 min	2 - 3	6 - 8
"	30 min	2 - 3	6 - 8
"	~1 h	2 - 5	6 - 8
"	~1 h	2 - 5	6 - 8
"	30 min	2 - 3	6 - 8
"	30 min	2 - 3	6 - 8

Classification and characteristics of insulins

(iii) Insulin mixtures (biphasic)			
Name	**Manufacturer**	**Structure**	**Vial, cartridge or pen**
Pre-mixed insulins			
Humalog Mix 25	Lilly	Analogue	Cartridge, pre-loaded pen
Humalog Mix 50	Lilly	Analogue	Cartridge, pre-loaded pen
Mixtard 30	Novo Nordisk	Human	Vial, cartridge, pre-loaded pen
Mixtard 10, 20, 40, 50	Novo Nordisk	Human	Cartridge, pre-loaded pen
Humulin M3	Lilly	Human	Vial, pre-loaded pen
Hypurin Porcine 30/70 mix	CP Pharmaceuticals	Pork	Vial, cartridge
Insuman comb 15	Aventis Pharma	Human	Pre-loaded pen
Insuman comb 25	Aventis Pharma	Human	Vial, cartridge, pre-loaded pen
Insuman comb 50	Aventis Pharma	Human	Cartridge, pre-loaded pen
NovoMix 30	Novo Nordisk	Analogue	Cartridge, pre-loaded pen
Pork Mixtard 30	Novo Nordisk	Pork	Vial

Fig 8.25

Timing of administration	Onset (min)	Peak (h)	Duration of action (h)
- 15 min before or during a meal	10	1 - 4	10 - 20
"	10	1 - 4	10 - 20
5 - 30 min before a meal	30	1 - 8	10 - 20
- 15 min before or during a meal	10	1 - 8	10 - 20
"	10	1 - 8	10 - 20
5 - 30 min before a meal	30	4 - 12	18 - 24
"	30	1 - 6	10 - 20
"	30	1 - 6	10 - 20
"	30	1 - 6	10 - 20
- 15 min before or during a meal	10	1 - 4	16 - 20
5 - 30 min before a meal	30	1 - 8	18 - 24

Diabetic ketoacidosis (DKA)

DKA management protocol	

Fluids

Various regimens have been proposed – some use colloid as well as crystalloid. Volume of fluid will alter according to degree of dehydration, age and comorbid factors.

1 litre	*In first ½ h*
1 litre	*Next 1 h*
1 litre	*Next 2 h*
1 litre	*Next 4 h*
2 - 5 litres	*In next 20 h*

Isotonic ('normal') saline (150 mmol/L)	*Generally used*
Hypotonic ('half-normal') saline (75 mmol/L)	*If plasma sodium >150 mmol/L*
5% glucose	*When blood glucose <15 mmol/L*
Sodium bicarbonate (600 ml of 1.26%)	*If pH <7.0*

Insulin

Continuous i.v. infusion

5 - 10 Units/h	*Initially*
2 - 4 Units/h maintenance (until able to eat)	*Titrated against blood glucose (measured hourly)*

Potassium

To each 1 litre of infused fluid

Add 40 mmol KCl	*If plasma K⁺ <3.5 mmol/L*
Add 20 mmol KCl	*If plasma K⁺ 3.5 - 5.5 mmol/L*
Add no KCl	*If plasma K⁺ >5.5 mmol/L*

Other measures

- Treat precipitating cause (e.g. infection, myocardial infarction).
- Hypotension should respond to adequate fluid replacement.
- Pass nasogastric tube if conscious level impaired.
- Adult respiratory distress syndrome – ventilation (100% O_2, IPPV).
- Cerebral oedema – consider i.v. mannitol or dexamethasone.
- Treat specific thromboembolic complications if they occur.

Fig 8.26

Diabetic hyperosmolar non-ketotic (HONK) state

HONK management protocol

Fluids

Volume of fluid will alter according to degree of dehydration, age and comorbid factors.

1 litre	*In first ½ h*
1 litre	*Next 1 h*
1 litre	*Next 2 h*

Then adjust according to requirements

Isotonic ('normal') saline (150 mmol/L)

Hypotonic ('half-normal') saline (75 mmol/L)   *If plasma sodium >150 mmol/L (no more than 1 - 2 litres)*

5% glucose   *When blood glucose <15 mmol/L*

Severely dehydrated patients need simultaneous saline infusion

Insulin

Continuous i.v. infusion

6 Units/h	*Initially – until blood glucose <15 mmol/L*
1 - 4 Units/h maintenance (until able to eat)	*Titrated against blood glucose (measured hourly)*

Potassium

To each 1 litre of infused fluid

Add 40 mmol KCl	*If plasma K⁺ <3.5 mmol/L*
Add 20 mmol KCl	*If plasma K⁺ 3.5 - 5.5 mmol/L*
Add no KCl	*If plasma K⁺ >5.5 mmol/L*

Other measures

- Treat precipitating cause (e.g. infection, myocardial infarction).
- Hypotension should respond to adequate fluid replacement.
- Pass nasogastric tube if conscious level impaired.
- Adult respiratory distress syndrome – ventilation (100% O_2, IPPV).
- Cerebral oedema – consider i.v. mannitol or dexamethasone.
- Routine use of low-dose heparin (thromboembolic complications are common).

Fig 8.27

Alpha-glucosidase inhibitor

Acarbose
Glucobay® (Bayer)

50 mg

100 mg

Sulphonylureas

Glibenclamide
non-proprietary (APS)

2.5 mg

5 mg

Gliclazide
Diamicron® (Servier)

80 mg

Gliclazide
non-proprietary (Alpharma)

80 mg

Gliclazide
Diamicron® MR (Servier)

30 mg

Glimepiride
Amaryl® (Aventis)

1 mg

2 mg

4 mg

Glipizide
non-proprietary (Pharmacia)

2.5 mg

non-proprietary (Norton)

5 mg

Tolbutamide
non-proprietary (Alpharma)

500 mg

Meglitinides

Repaglinide
NovoNorm® (Novo Nordisk)

1 mg

2 mg

Nateglinide
Starlix® (Novartis)

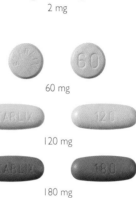

60 mg

120 mg

180 mg

Biguanide

Metformin
Glucophage® (Merck)

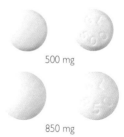

500 mg

850 mg

Metformin
Glucophage SR® (Merck)

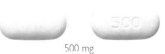

500 mg

Thiazolidinediones

Pioglitazone
Actos® (Takeda)

15 mg

30 mg

Rosiglitazone
Avandia® (GSK)

4 mg

8 mg

Combination

Rosiglitazone-metformin
Avandamet® (GSK)

1 mg rosiglitazone
500 mg metformin

2 mg rosiglitazone
500 mg metformin

Injection devices

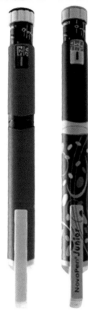
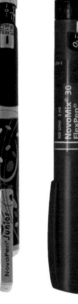
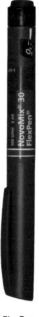
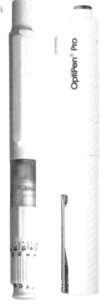

NovoPen3   **NovoPen Junior**   **FlexPen**   **OptiSet**   **OptiPen® Pro**

Pens in upper panel shown at half actual size.

Devices in lower panel shown at one-third actual size.

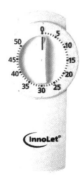
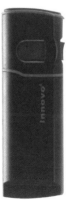

InnoLet   **Innovo**

Insulin syringes

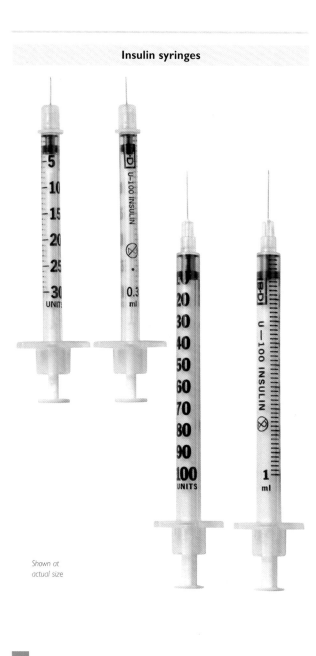

*Shown at
actual size*

Insulins

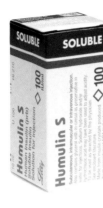
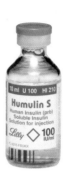

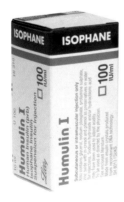
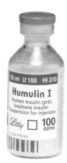

Insulins

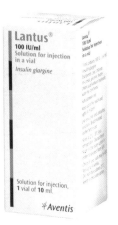

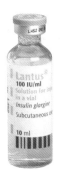

Lantus®
100 IU/ml
Solution for injection
in a vial

Insulin glargine

Solution for injection,
1 vial of 10 ml.

✢ **Aventis**

Lantus®
100 IU/ml
**Solution for injection
in a cartridge**

Insulin glargine

Subcutaneous use.
This cartridge is for use in conjunction with OptiPen®.

Solution for injection,
5 cartridges of **3** ml

✢ **Aventis**

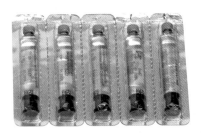

Insulins

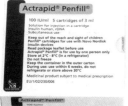

Actrapid® Penfill®

100 IU/ml   5 cartridges of 3 ml
Solution for injection in a cartridge
Insulin human, rDNA
Subcutaneous use

Keep out of the reach and sight of children
Penfill® cartridges for use with Novo Nordisk
insulin devices
Read package leaflet before use
Actrapid® Penfill® is for use by one person only
Store at 2°C - 8°C (in a refrigerator)
Do not freeze
Keep the container in the outer carton
During use: use within 6 weeks, do not
refrigerate or store above 30°C

Medicinal product subject to medical prescription

EU/1/02/230/006

Actrapid® Penfill®
100 IU/ml

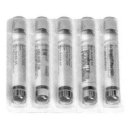

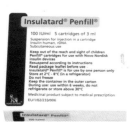

Insulatard® Penfill®

100 IU/ml   5 cartridges of 3 ml
Suspension for injection in a cartridge
Insulin human, rDNA
Subcutaneous use

Keep out of the reach and sight of children
Penfill® cartridges for use with Novo Nordisk
insulin devices
Resuspend according to instructions
Read package leaflet before use
Insulatard® Penfill® is for use by one person only
Store at 2°C - 8°C (in a refrigerator)
Do not freeze
Keep the container in the outer carton
During use: use within 6 weeks, do not
refrigerate or store above 30°C

Medicinal product subject to medical prescription

EU/1/02/233/006

Insulatard® Penfill®
100 IU/ml

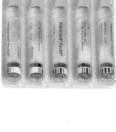

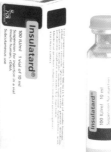

Insulatard®

100 IU/ml   1 vial of 10 ml
Suspension for injection in a vial
Insulin human, rDNA
Subcutaneous use

Insulins

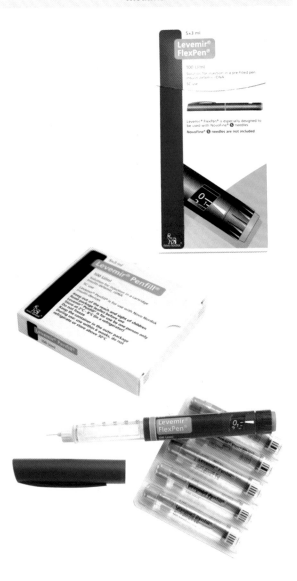

SELECTED READING

Books

Textbook of diabetes, 3rd edn. Pickup JC, Williams G (eds). Blackwell, Oxford, 2003.

International textbook of diabetes mellitus, 3rd edn. DeFronzo RA, Ferrannini E, Keen H, Zimmet P (eds). Wiley, Chichester, 2004.

Diabetes mellitus, 2nd edn. Campbell IW, Lebovitz H. Health Press, Oxford, 2001.

Type 2 diabetes in practice. Krentz AJ, Bailey CJ. Roy Soc Med Press, London, 2001.

Therapy for diabetes mellitus and related disorders, 4th edn. Lebovitz H (ed). American Diabetes Association, Alexandria VA, 2004.

Guidelines

A desktop guide to type 2 diabetes mellitus. European Diabetes Policy Group 1998 - 1999. *Diabetic Medicine* 1999; **16**: 716-730.

Management of type 2 diabetes. Clinical guideline G. Management of blood glucose. National Institute for Clinical Excellence, London 2002, 19pp.

Standards of medical care in diabetes. Position statement: American Diabetes Association. *Diabetes Care* 2004; **27**: suppl 1, S15-S35.

Reviews

Bailey CJ, Day C. Antidiabetic drugs. *Br J Cardiol* 2003; **10**: 128-136.

Feher MD, Bailey CJ. Reclassifying insulins. *Br J Diabetes Vasc Dis* 2004; **4**: 39-42.

Inzucchi SE. Oral antihyperglycemic therapy for type 2 diabetes. *JAMA* 2002; **287**: 360-372.

DeFronzo RA. Pharmacologic therapy for type 2 diabetes mellitus. *Ann Intern Med* 1999; **131**: 281-303.

Lebovitz HE. Alpha-glucosidase inhibitors as agents in the treatment of diabetes. *Diabetes Rev* 1998; **6**: 132-145.

Lebovitz HE. Insulin secretagogues: old and new. *Diabetes Rev* 1999; **7**: 139-153.

Dornhorst A. Insulinotropic meglitinide analogues. *Lancet* 2001; **358**: 1709-1716.

Bailey CJ, Turner RC. Metformin. *N Engl J Med* 1996; **334**: 577-579.

Bailey CJ, Day C. Thiazolidinediones. *Br J Diabetes Vasc Dis* 2000; **1**: 7-13.

Barnett AH. A review of basal insulins. *Diabetic Medicine* 2003; **20**: 873-885.

Barnett AH, Owens DR. Insulin analogues. *Lancet* 1997; **349**: 47-51.

Bolli GB, Owens DR. Insulin glargine. *Lancet* 2000; **356**: 443-445.

Index